VALUE CONFLICTS IN
HEALTH CARE DELIVERY

VALUE CONFLICTS IN
HEALTH CARE DELIVERY

Edited by

BART GRUZALSKI
CARL NELSON

BALLINGER PUBLISHING COMPANY
Cambridge, Massachusetts
A Subsidiary of Harper & Row, Publishers, Inc.

International Standard Book Number: 0-88410-735-3

Library of Congress Catalog Card Number: 82-3896

Printed in the United States of America

Library of Congress Cataloging in Publication Data

Main entry under title:

Value conflicts in health care delivery.

   Includes index.
   1. Medical ethics—Address, essays, lectures.
I. Gruzalski, Bart. II. Nelson, Carl Ellis, 1916-
[DNLM: 1. Ethics, Medical. 2. Philosophy, Medical.
3. Delivery of health care. W 61 V215]
R724.V33   174'.2   82-3896
ISBN 0-88410-735-3

To Our Parents

CONTENTS

PREFACE

Although we originally set out to understand the sources and dimensions of contemporary value conflicts in health care delivery, it immediately became clear that we were less interested in viewing moral puzzles as they arose in specific cases than in viewing them in the context of the mainstream of economic, political, and social thought. We reasoned that the likelihood of resolving value conflicts would be enhanced by an interdisciplinary viewpoint. Moreover, since the audience we wished to reach included patients, providers, administrators, ethicists, and others, we sought to invite contributions from scholars and practitioners who were comfortable with the blurred lines that typify the features of moral dilemmas as they arise in health care delivery.

The collaborative effort between the two editors of this volume parallels the interdisciplinary process we believe is necessary for dealing with medical-ethical problems. As educators in two divergent disciplines, we literally found ourselves with limitations of common language, perspective, and purpose. The practicality governing the thinking of a person trained in administration contrasts with the analytical methods of inquiry of someone trained in twentieth century philosophy. As a first organizing principle, we discussed and agreed upon a working list of fundamental value conflicts that dominate health care delivery. The list ranged from problems in the definition of health to questions of allocation, equity, paternalism, and autonomy. Where possible, and based upon our own backgrounds, we then tried to illustrate each area of conflict by specific examples. Having framed the problems, we set out to identify those individuals who were known for their informed and sometimes controversial positions and who would be able to present their ideas to a general audience. (Six of the chapters in this volume were presented as part of Northeastern University's Health Care Colloquium Series, which we codirect.) Our final group of contributors includes individuals with advanced degrees in medicine, philosophy, law, and administration, most of whom are known in academic circles throughout the United States and abroad.

As the project progressed, we regretted the omission of some viewpoints, notably, economics, medical sociology, anthropology, and political science. Nevertheless, the fact that many of our contributors regularly cross academic boundaries, while others practice in an amalgam of disciplines, convinces us that our interdisciplinary mission has not been sacrificed. Although one alternative in any decisionmaking process is to seek more information, the search should stop at the point where the added cost of searching begins to exceed the expected value of additional information. In the interests of producing a short, readable collection of original essays, we believe we have come close to that ideal.

For some readers, projects like ours that encourage pluralistic viewpoints and possibly dissent in an area (medicine) manifestly based upon positivistic scientific methods may be disquieting. Too much pluralism, they argue, will lead to disarray, delay, higher costs, and a diminution of faith essential to the caring process. This argument loses validity, however, when it is realized that medicine does not exist beyond the context of cultures, politics, and personalities, that medicine is always practiced under conditions of uncertainty, and that medicine itself is a social response to patient complaints that may never fall neatly under the categories of medical science. Others may welcome a pluralistic approach for the equally objectionable reason that it can serve as a means for evading personal responsibility. The physician or administrator who gains comfort, peace of mind, and legal protection by hiding behind a consent form or an ethics committee to avoid responsibility or disguise incompetence cannot be excused. Physicians and administrators have their own personal and professional responsibilities, and if an ethics committee condones what a physician or administrator believes to be wrong, those responsibilities create an even greater and more complex burden for the physician or administrator.

In this book we are not concerned with what values are, but rather with how they come into conflict and how these conflicts may be resolved. As a result, we want to encourage participants in medical decisionmaking to contemplate the values implied by their actions and how such values may come into conflict with different values they or others hold. Some might argue, for example, that health should be the overriding value since the absence of health threatens our ability to enjoy other values. Others might quickly question how much autonomy, honesty, comfort, or control one may be willing to give up to achieve or gamble for improved health. Still others may question whether the individual's interests are more important than the interests of the family, society, or science. There is, in addition, a range of opinions as to what health, health care, and health care delivery should encompass, and these diverse opinions are at the core of many medical-ethical and policy dilemmas—they serve as one starting point for an informed dialogue.

A pluralistic and interdisciplinary approach to these questions accepts the reality that assessments and valuations by participants in the health care process are often in flux. Received values are continually tested and challenged by developments in medical diagnosis, treatment, and by shifts in the organization of the delivery system, and value conflicts emerge from the interplay of forces inside and outside of the medical domain. Only a pluralistic interdisciplinary approach is appropriate to the new and extraordinarily difficult bioethical problems that accompany these changes. As society and individuals gain knowledge and fluctuate between conflicting values that may not be capable of simultaneous satisfaction, we should expect increased confusion and controversy. Permanent or temporary resolution of these problems requires broad-based skills and the participation of experts and lay persons with a variety of viewpoints. Since values are the product of historical and cultural development and are based upon desires, expectations, and experience, there can be no formal calculus other than open discussion for establishing guidelines for action. A pluralistic approach carries the minimal guarantee that all parties will be heard, and that in itself may be all we are capable of achieving.

The thirteen contributions in this volume share a common concern for the pluralistic exploration of values in health care delivery and, as a result, demonstrate convincingly that ethical issues in health care not only include but extend beyond the currently fashionable dialogue over patient rights. In Part I, "Scope and Origins of Some Value Conflicts in Health Care Delivery," the authors focus upon the definition of health and illness and the role of medicine by considering the province and goals of medicine from historical, epistemological, and normative perspectives. As a unit, the chapters in this section demonstrate the extraordinary power medicine has over our lives and how this came to be so. The primary source of value conflict here is one of marking the appropriate sphere for medical involvement, control, and responsibility. In Part II, "Confronting Ethical Issues," the authors discuss various arenas in which medical-ethical issues arise and the rights and responsibilities of the parties to these dilemmas. The essays here are process oriented, providing guidelines and limitations for patients, providers, lawyers, and bioethicists. In Part III, "Cooperative Methods For Resolving Value Conflicts in Health Care," the authors exemplify the interdisciplinary efforts we believe are essential to resolving contemporary value conflicts confronting patients, patient advocates, and health care providers. Whether these conflicts arise at the individual patient or policy assessment level, a diversity of viewpoints and open dialogue should ultimately clarify issues and guarantee pluralistically based resolutions that will provide guidance in the day-by-day delivery of health care.

Medicine will continue to influence and be influenced by changes in values occurring throughout our society. As participants in these developments—as patients, physicians, nurses, philosophers, administrators, or concerned observers—our primary task is to be aware of conflicts of value when they arise and to join in the dialogue they engender. If our book sparks a spirit of pluralistic cooperation toward the resolution of value conflicts by exposing individuals to the virtues of this approach, then as authors we will gain some assurance of the value of our own efforts. The book's ultimate value, however, depends upon the changes it brings to the delivery of health services and to the activities of everyone concerned.

Bart Gruzalski
Carl Nelson

ACKNOWLEDGMENTS

This collection of essays developed because of our work as codirectors of Northeastern University's Interdisciplinary Faculty Health Care Colloquium Series and the generous support of the Northeastern University Provost's Office. We are especially indebted to Gerald Herman, who as Special Assistant to the Provost for Faculty Development encouraged us from the inception of this project and was instrumental in our receiving necessary financial assistance. Without his help this project would not have come about, and we are deeply grateful to him. We also very gratefully acknowledge the direct participatory support of Melvin Mark, Provost and Senior Vice President of Academic Affairs, Philip Crotty, Vice Provost, Karl Weiss, Vice Provost, Arthur Smith, Associate Provost, Patricia Hinds, Assistant to the Provost, and Suzanne Geetter, former Assistant to the Provost, each of whom not only encouraged us but actively helped out with a number of the private and public duties that are part of any university colloquium series.

We want to give special thanks to Samuel Gorovitz of the University of Maryland who not only was our first speaker and contributor, but who provided us with valuable guidance along the way. We also want to give special thanks to George Annas of the Boston University School of Medicine for his early support of our series, for twice participating in our colloquia, and for suggesting potential contributors to this volume. In addition we thank the other individuals who acted as discussants for the colloquia of our contributors, and they include Richard Daynard, Suzanne Greenberg, Morris Horowitz, Keith Howell, and Irene Nichols, all of Northeastern University, and Daryl B. Matthews, of Boston University Medical School. For his assistance in providing needed documents, we also thank Dwight Blankenbaker of the National Center for Health Care Technology. Finally, we are pleased to express our thanks to Sharon B. Young for her support and helpful suggestions as this project developed.

We thank the editors of the *Annals of Internal Medicine* for permission to include the article by James L. Bernat, Charles M. Culver, and Bernard Gert, the editors of the *Einstein Quarterly* for permission to include the forthcoming essay by Ruth Macklin, and the editors of Prentice-Hall for permission to include much of the last chapter of Andrew Jameton's forthcoming volume, *Nursing Ethics: The Practice of Nursing and the Moral Problems of Health Care.* Finally, although it may not be customary for coeditors to acknowledge publicly the assistance that each provided to the efforts of the other, we would be remiss without recognizing the mutual respect and gratitude we hold for one another's total contribution to this joint endeavor.

B. G.

C. N.

I SCOPE AND ORIGINS OF VALUE CONFLICTS IN HEALTH CARE DELIVERY

Almost every controversy in medical ethics involves the concepts of health and disease. But what is health? What is disease? Should a "psychotic" murderer be treated as a sick person or be punished as a criminal? Is a patient *sick* who complains of pain although a physician can find no corresponding pathological condition? Related to the controversy over the concepts of health and disease is the practical issue of what conditions medicine and health care providers are to treat. For example, if an elderly person is saved from starving to death and is then sent home, is the maintenance of an adequate diet a medical concern? Does sex education have anything to do with the practice of medicine? Should institutions take into consideration the wishes of patients and families in scheduling surgeries? Do physicians have a professional responsibility to work to prevent nuclear war? These and a host of similar issues trouble health care providers, lawmakers, bioethicists, and others who are concerned with the scope of medicine, medical responsibility, and the corresponding economic and political issues that affect all of our lives. The following five chapters focus on the important array of problems that deal with the scope and limits of medicine and medical responsibility.

In "The Concept of Psychosis: A Cause and a Consequence of Certain Medical-Ethical Dilemmas" Thomas Szasz argues that there is a dilemma at the foundations of psychiatry. On the one hand, the

1

model for medical disease is the objective pathological lesion. On the other hand, psychosis—*the* "disease" of the "medicine" of psychiatry—is not defined in terms of lesions but rather in moral and legal terms, viz., bad behavior and legal irresponsibility. Hence, as Szasz concludes, "the moral judgment and power relations that psychiatry has banished from its perception . . . thus return via the back door." Underlying this dilemma is psychosis, which, according to Thomas Szasz, is a very different condition from what people ordinarily think it is. According to Szasz, when psychosis is not a hidden brain disease, it is in fact a form of dishonesty participated in by both patient and doctor. The dishonesty involves an imitation and some role play (e.g., pretending that one is following the dictates of a Secret Voice and playing out this pretense). Both patient and doctor participate in not holding the patient responsible for his or her bad behavior during the role play, and the participation of each is what legitimizes the role of the other. Szasz closes his provocative essay by explicitly raising the question upon which his and the following two essays focus: What counts as a disease? The answer Szasz suggests is that only pathological conditions are diseases, and this view is defended in the chapter which follows.

John Ladd begins his chapter "The Concepts of Health and Disease and Their Ethical Implications" by defining a disease as a verifiable pathological condition. On the basis of this definition, he argues that the proper province of medicine is only the treatment, cure, and prevention of diseases, and *not* the wider concerns of health and health care. According to Ladd, identifying a lack of disease with health has produced the overmedicalization of American society, and he cites several consequences of this overmedicalization: staggering costs of medical care, our society's obsession with health and medical problems, too many problems being laid on the laps of physicians, and, in general, the treatment of social problems (e.g., alcoholism, drug addiction, and teenage pregnancy) as medical problems requiring medical treatment in pursuit of medical cures. Ladd's suggestion is that by being clearer about the differences between the categories of health and disease we may avoid some of these consequences. Although Ladd is certainly correct in arguing that many problems not involving pathological conditions do not need to be treated as medical problems, the important question is whether they may properly fall within the domain of medicine. Consider Ladd's example of teenage pregnancy. Might not this problem have medical ramifications, particularly if the pregnant teenager wants or needs an abortion? Or consider the prevention of teenage pregnancy: Is it out of the domain of medicine to inform young people about the risks and benefits of birth control and to develop birth control devices? Would taking this issue completely out of the medical domain be advantageous? Whatever one thinks about these and related issues, Ladd's narrow definition of the scope of medicine and medical care sharpens important questions that the next three authors critically examine.

In contrast to Ladd, Tristram Engelhardt claims that limiting the domain of medicine only to the verifiably pathological would be unwholesome because it would lead to discounting patient complaints that do not readily match up with verifiable lesions—yet medicine developed *precisely* to deal with those problems that manifested themselves as patient complaints. The overemphasis of the pathophysical leads to anomalies like the claim that the operation was a success but the patient died. In "The Subordination of the Clinic" Engelhardt shows that medicine through the eighteenth century was so focused on patient complaints that diseases were catalogued *in terms of* these complaints. The revolution during the eighteenth and nineteenth centuries toward viewing diseases as pathoanatomical and pathophysiological changes within the body has, of course, provided medicine with reliable explanatory and predictive accounts that helped in the prevention, cure, and amelioration of illness. But underlying this revolution in the classification of disease is always the patient complaint, and hence, according to Engelhardt, to limit the domain of medicine only to the verifiable lesion would be to forget the point of this social enterprise. Engelhardt does not deny that there are boundaries between religion, education, medicine, and so on, but argues that these boundaries overlap. Problems of alcoholism, for example, might be claimed by all three, as might also be problems with teenage pregnancy. The moral is that physicians should not forget that medicine developed its technology to better treat patient complaints, and, hence, the practice of medicine should include being responsive to patient complaints even if they do not correspond to objectively verifiable pathophysical conditions.

The focus on patient complaints, values, and concerns is further developed in Carl Nelson's "Time and Health Care Delivery." In his chapter Nelson sharply distinguishes between clock or "objective" time and personal or "subjective" time. The twentieth century focus on verifiable lesions is consistent with the focus of contemporary medicine on objective or clock time. Yet is is precisely the focus on clock time that leads to many value conflicts between patients, upon whom clock time is imposed, and the medical institution, in which clock time is the norm. In the three areas of kidney dialysis, the scheduling of surgeries, and health prevention, Nelson identifies value conflicts that arise because of differences between the clock time imposed by institutions and the subjective time of the patient. In each area Nelson suggests several possible ways in which these conflicts might be resolved to the benefit of both the patient and the health care providers. For example, in the scheduling of surgeries, institutions typically respond to the preferences of surgeons, medical staff, and, finally, to random orderings. Nelson argues that an appropriate ethical position would require also giving weight to patient preferences that are not trivial, and this, of course, requires systematic investigations ending in a collaborative judgment that takes all the relevant preferences into consideration. Nelson concludes that health care providers should take the preferences of patients into account in order to consider the patient as a whole person, not merely as the site of a disease.

In "The Last Epidemic: Medical Responsibility and Thermonuclear War" Andrew Jameton and Christine Cassel argue that physicians have a central and urgent moral responsibility to work to prevent nuclear war. The conclusion of their persuasive argument places a special responsibility on physicians and bioethicists to do what we can to participate in the antinuclear war movement. That, in fact, is one reason why we included their essay in this volume, although during the period since we decided to include the essay much happened in the antinuclear war movement: demonstrations erupted in Europe, the movement gained strength in the United States, and, significantly, the American Medical Association endorsed the position to prevent nuclear war advocated by Physicians for Social Responsibility.

But there is also a second reason why we included Jameton and Cassel's essay in the opening section. Insofar as their central argument is sound, it follows that the practice of medicine not only includes the treatment of verifiable lesions and a caring response to patient complaints, but also imposes on physicians the responsibility to participate in enterprises that are crucial for the prevention of diseases that would be difficult to treat once they began. It also follows that the proper domain of medicine and medical responsibility is much broader than is usually thought. One only has to consider the medical warning against cigarette smoking and the medical advice to exercise regularly to see that medicine has a proper function in a wide arena of social activities. In short, the scope of medicine overlaps the scope of religion, politics, and law, and the responsibilities of health care providers overlap the responsibilities of those engaged in these and other social enterprises.

1 THE CONCEPT OF PSYCHOSIS
A Cause and a Consequence of Certain Medical-Ethical Dilemmas

Thomas Szasz

ILLNESS AND IRRESPONSIBILITY

In December 1976 Roxanne Gay killed her husband, Blenda, a defensive end on the Philadelphia Eagles professional football team, by plunging a knife into his throat while he was asleep. Witnesses at her trial testified that she "suffered from hallucinations that her husband, her family, and the police were plotting to kill her."[1] Mrs. Gay was acquitted as not guilty by reason of insanity and was committed to the Marlboro State Psychiatric Hospital in New Jersey.

On July 31, 1980, Camden (New Jersey) County Judge I.V. DiMartino ordered that Mrs. Gay be released because she "has achieved that degree of mental stability where she is no longer a danger to herself, her family, or society." In a telephone interview with the *New York Times*, Judge DiMartino added: "She has had a complete remission of her psychotic episodes and several psychiatrists testified that continuation of her hospitalization would be detrimental."[2]

This news item, which is typical of stories that appear nearly every day in our newspapers and magazines, tells us what a "psychosis" really is in a way in that neither Webster's dictionary nor psychiatric textbooks do. Webster's defines psychosis as "mental disease; any serious mental derangement"; psychiatric texts speak similarly of "severe mental diseases." Who would suspect what lurks behind this facile medical rhetoric? In particular, who would suspect that the operational meaning of "psychosis"—the meaning that we can infer from its actual use—refers in part to the criminal nonresponsibility of the person afflicted with this alleged malady and in part to the person's committability as an involuntary patient to a mental hospital? In short, who would suspect that the idea of psychosis *justifies* exculpating the guilty as "not guilty" (by reason of insanity) and inculpating the innocent as "dangerous" (by reason of insanity)?

Ordinary bodily diseases, like peptic ulcer or cancer of the liver, are defined in terms of *lesions*, that is, in pathological terms. But psychosis—with schizophrenia as its paradigm—is defined in terms of *lack of responsibility*, that is, in moral and legal terms.

Responsibility and nonresponsibility are, of course, ethical concepts. In our society, not all persons are considered to be responsible; for example, the very young, the very old or senile, and certain brain damaged persons are regarded as not rational and hence not responsible. (Most societies make some such distinction between those regarded as rational/responsible and those regarded as irrational/not responsible.)

Introducing the concept of rationality into this discussion provides some empirical foundation for the judgments with which we are confronted. Some people never develop the normal use of some of their body parts and functions. For example, the congenitally blind person cannot see; similarly, infants cannot use their muscles to support themselves or their brains to think "rationally." Others lose the use of certain bodily functions. For example, the person in congestive heart failure has a failing heart and the person with senile dementia has a failing brain.

Although the irrationality of dementia is just as objective and observable as is the immobility of a person disabled by severe arthritis, there is a difference between them: the mobility or immobility of a joint is a biological standard, whereas the rationality or irrationality of reasoning or thinking is a personal or societal standard. We thus ascertain whether someone is "rational" (or "oriented") by determining whether the person knows who and where he or she is, who the President is, and so forth. There is nothing wrong with this standard. What is wrong is that psychiatry conflates and confuses the irrationality of *dementia* with the irrationality of *psychosis*. The former is a symptom of a malfunctioning *brain*, whereas the latter is not.[3]

If a psychosis is not the symptom of a hidden (as yet undiagnosed or undiagnosable) brain disease, then what is it? The answer is, I am afraid, too simple: It is a form of behavior. More specifically, it is behavior judged to be *bad*—injurious to the self or others. It is also a form of behavior closely connected with the actor's dishonesty: a person who is honest with others, and especially with himself, cannot be or become psychotic. (Such a person may, of course, be called psychotic by others.)

RATIONALITY AND RESPONSIBILITY

Wherein lies the essential difference between the irrationality of a demented person and of a psychotic one? The demented person *displays a defect*—typically of memory (he cannot remember the date or even who he is) and of his ability to reason (he cannot do simple arithmetical tasks that he could easily do formerly). The psychotic person, on the other hand, *asserts a false claim*—typically of his identity (he is Jesus or God) and of his reasons for having engaged in acts injurious to himself or others (he acted on the command of God or demons or in self-defense against nonexisting persecutors).

For example, Roxanne Gay, with whose story I began this chapter, claimed not only insanity but also that she killed her husband because she was a "battered wife." Several experts testified at her trial that there was no evidence that her husband had beaten her. Characteristically, the *Times* referred to her false claims as "hallucinations." The point is that we do not now consider being beaten by one's husband as an excuse for killing him, but we do so consider being psychotic.

How, then, do we ascertain a particular person who has committed a violent act was or was not psychotic? The answer is: We don't. That is the wrong question to ask. The right question is: Under what circumstances do we *ascribe* psychosis to the perpetrator of a certain act? The answer to this question tells us a good deal about the true nature of "psychosis." However, before considering this question, let us consider briefly the question of the ascription of responsibility, with which we are more familiar.

A 5-year-old is not criminally responsible for killing people in a housefire that he has started by playing with matches. But his mother or father may hold him responsible for not washing his hands before a meal and may punish him for it. Without going into the details of this complex concept, let us note only that when we say that a person "acts responsibly," we usually mean that he acts with *care*. A man is considered to be responsible if he takes good care of himself and of other people, that is, if he acts dependably and safely. If he endangers others—for example, if he drinks too much or is a spendthrift—he may be called an "irresponsible father," a phrase by which we do not, however, mean to exonerate him from being a bad father. In such a case, most of us follow the Sartrean principle of holding that a person "is responsible for being irresponsible." That statement may sound like a contradiction, but it isn't: The term "irresponsible" functions here merely as a way of expressing our disapproval of a particular behavior.

We also use the term "irresponsible" (or "not responsible") to conceal our strategy toward the person so designated, as exemplified in the courtroom scenarios where defendants are "acquitted" as not guilty because not responsible, because of insanity. Here the term functions as a vehicle for our judgment that he should be handled differently from persons deemed to be responsible.

One more observation concerning the ascription of responsibility and its implication for the authorities' strategy toward the agent in question must be mentioned here. Although we do not usually regard animals as moral agents, we often treat them—especially domestic and circus animals—as if they were responsible for their actions. We reward them for good deeds and punish them for bad, even executing them when they kill. When a pet German shepherd mauls a child or when a circus elephant tramples his trainer, the "guilty" animal is often put to death. This example illustrates the conflation of the descriptive and dispositive meanings of the term "responsibility": The animal was "responsible" for killing a human being, and its "responsibility" justifies our killing him. Since we believe that we must not punish agents not responsible for their acts, we must, if we still wish to control them, either "find" them to be responsible, as we do the animals mentioned, or "punish" them by nonpunitive ("therapeutic") means, as we do persons diagnosed as psychotic.

PSYCHOSIS AS SELF-JUSTIFICATION

It may be objected that I dwell unduly on the issue of responsibility as a crucial parameter of psychosis. But the plain facts about this alleged illness, as against the rhetoric in which it is couched and the theories by which it is ostensibly explained, fully justify this emphasis. What are these facts?

Typically, a diagnosis of psychosis is made when two conditions obtain: The first condition is that, by conventional standards, a person behaves badly, often very badly; the second one is that the person then justifies the behavior in a conventionally unjustifiable way—typically, by claiming that what he has done is not bad but good. Examples abound in the daily press:

Willie Robinson, 42, was placed under "police protection" at the Wesson Unit of Bay State Medical Center [in Springfield, Mass.] yesterday [June 23, 1980], a short time after he allegedly went berserk with a long-bladed kitchen knife in the crowded waiting room of the hospital's Springfield Unit. . . . [At the hospital], Robinson assaulted the guard and several women and allegedly pinned a [six-year-old] boy to the ground near an ambulance entrance and stabbed him repeatedly screaming, 'I'm the king! I'm the king! Now I've done it. I'm done.' [The boy died.][4]

A Roxdale [Ontario] woman signed her husband out of a psychiatric ward against medical advice days before he stabbed her 58 times in front of their three children, an Ontario Supreme Court jury heard yesterday. . . . William Szeman, 41, pleaded not guilty yesterday [June 26, 1980] to second degree murder by reason of insanity. Lawyers on both sides of the case . . . agreed that Mr. Szeman should be found insane. The insanity finding needed only the jury's official approval and that took less than 15 minutes. . . . The jury was told that Mr. Szeman, an auto body worker who came to Canada from Hungary in 1957, was admitted to the psychiatric ward of Etobicoke General Hospital last April 18, three days before the murder [sic]. Metro Police Sergeant Donald Sampson testified that . . . Mr. Szeman told him he worked with Germans, Hungarians, and Poles who hated him because he had fought against them during the last world war. Mr. Szeman would have been 7 when the war ended. . . . Mr. William Peacock [a neighbor] said that Mr. Szeman, walking by him after his arrest, said: 'She was trying to poison me.' There is no evidence that was true. . . .[5]

The pattern so obvious in the behavior of these and other like-minded malefactors, yet so systematically neglected in psychiatric theorizing about them, has several significant features:

1. The "patient" engages in highly destructive acts, often severely injuring or killing people, as in both of the above cases.
2. The "patient" makes false claims about himself: that he is a king, in the first case; that he fought in the Second World War and was being poisoned by his wife, in the second.
3. The "patient" justifies what he has done—as self-defense (against being poisoned) or a "right" (as king or god).
4. The "patient" feels relieved by his act and exults in it. In the first case, the killer exclaimed: "Now I've done it. I'm done." In the second, he was found "prancing and dancing near the body of his wife, which lay on the pavement in the driveway."[6]

Clearly, the standard psychiatric explanation, which attributes such "berserk" acts to an acute, overwhelming disorder of the brain rendering the "patient" irrational and violent, cannot account for any of these features. In particular, it cannot account for why the "patient" feels proud rather than ashamed of what he has done. In the language of the McNaghten's Rule, the oldest Anglo–American test of criminal insanity, such malefactors are said not to know right from wrong. But this is patently not true: in fact, they keep insisting on *their judgments of right and wrong.* What the evidence thus points to is not their inability to judge right from wrong, but their inversion of our judgments of right and wrong.

The attempt to explain psychosis medically faces still another serious difficulty, which can be summed up in the following question: Why does the hypothetical brain disease causing psychosis always manifest itself in dramatically bad behavior rather than in dramatically good behavior? Why do "psychotic patients" attack and kill people rather than assist and help them? The answer, as I see it, is because good acts or good behavior would not accomplish the purposes that motivate the psychotic. This answer, as we shall see, also helps to explain what "is" a psychosis.

PSYCHOSIS AS SELF-DRAMATIZATION

Like all human behavior, so-called psychotic behavior may have a variety of motivations. Many such acts, such as those illustrated by the stories I have cited, are inspired by an intense desire for attention and fame in a person who can accomplish that goal in no other way than through a dramatic act of violence. Such an act and its aftermath also satisfy the actor's intense desire for being distracted from his own insignificance, from the drudgery and ordinariness of his everyday life and its frustrations; in short, from the bleakness and pointlessness of his life.

Psychosis, then, has this in common with war (and also with dramatic criminality): Each provides a surpassingly successful distraction from everyday problems—psychosis for the individual, war (and revolution) for the masses. This interpretation is consistent with the seemingly paradoxical sense of inner peace that "psychotics" experience after their "acute episode" of mayhem and that "normal" people experience after being "mobilized" for revolution or war.

The so-called psychotic thus replaces a life filled with emptiness and boredom with a life filled with drama and excitement. Nowhere is this more evident than in cases of so-called paranoia or paranoid schizophrenia—behavior patterns that are, in fact, the caricatures of detective stories. In these "clinicalized" whodunits, "patients" cast themselves—alternately or sometimes even simultaneously—in the dual roles of utterly helpless victims and all-powerful agents. And all this is wrapped, as I suggested earlier, in a transparent but fashionable sheath of deceit.

What I am suggesting is that psychotic behavior is an impersonation or act, as in a play. "All the world's a stage, and all the men and women merely players," said Shakespeare: a perspective that applies with special force to so-called psychotics. The famous case of the "Son of Sam" is an instructive example.

The "Son of Sam" was a young man named David Berkowitz who terrorized New York City in 1976 and 1977 by killing six people and wounding seven others. At the time of his trial, Berkowitz justified the killings by claiming that he was carrying out the orders of demons and a dog. Barely eighteen months later, in an effort to scuttle a multimillion-dollar book and movie project about him and his crime, Berkowitz claimed that his crazy behavior was an act. Speaking to an Associated Press reporter in Attica (New York) prison, Berkowitz said of the stories he told after being arrested: "Quite frankly, this is fictitious, it is invented, it is a lie. There were no real demons, no talking dogs, no Satanic henchmen. I made it all up."[7]

Confronted with Berkowitz's claim that he was faking insanity, Dr. Daniel Schwartz, who headed a team of doctors that examined Berkowitz and testified that he was psychotic, said that if "it [the story of demonic possession] was an act, it was an all-time winner." He explained that he believed Berkowitz's story because it was "so convincing and had so much peripheral validation."[8] That, of course, is nonsense. Schwartz accepted the "Son of Sam" story because by legitimizing Berkowitz as "psychotic" he was legitimizing himself as a psychiatrist.

In August 1980 Berkowitz gave an interview to the *Buffalo Evening News* reiterating his plea that he "is not now and never was mentally ill. . . . Bearded now and noticeably thinner than in 1977, he insists he was not mentally ill when he was in the Army, not when he was firing a gun at nameless faces in New York's dark lovers' lanes, not when he was being examined by psychiatrists and not when he was screaming out in the courtroom."[9] The reporter who interviewed Berkowitz noted that "Berkowitz acted like a sane man. And he talked like a sane man." But then he added the characteristic caveat of our age: "Yet what is one to think of someone who for no visible reason shot at 15 people he didn't know, killing six of them, injuring seven, and missing two?"[10] The implication of this question, to which I shall return presently, is that anyone who acts this way is, and must be, crazy, mentally ill, psychotic.

Some of the things Berkowitz told the *Buffalo Evening News* reporter are worth mentioning here. "The tapes," Berkowitz explained, "are authentic in that I said those things [demons impelling him to kill, etc.], but they are not authentic because I was feigning and malingering."[11] Berkowitz said he was faking insanity to allay his guilt for the killings. Perhaps so, in part. But I believe he was doing so for the added dramatic attention his claims assured him. In any case, Berkowitz is not petitioning the courts for a hearing to declare him competent to manage his affairs; he had been declared incompetent and assigned a conservator to manage his affairs. "Paramount to Berkowitz's current plans," according to the *Buffalo Evening News*, "is a court's recognition that he is sane. If clear, articulate responses and conversation coupled with normal amounts of smiling and laughter and the appreciation of nuances and good and evil concepts are signs of competency, then David Berkowitz is all there."[12]

The reporter's judgment of Berkowitz's sanity is supported by the judgments of the prison personnel who, according to Berkowitz, will testify for him. Says Frances Mills, chief of psychiatric services at the Attica Correctional Facility, who sees Berkowitz almost daily: "I have never found him psychotic."[13] Another Attica official described Berkowitz as "crazy as a fox"[14]—illustrating that a homely phrase might tell us more about "psychosis" than a shelf-full of psychiatric textbooks. Although Berkowitz now acknowledges that his crimes were "horrendous" and "despicable," and although he is serving a 315-year prison sentence and is offering fresh and convincing evidence of not being psychotic, he is, nevertheless, receiving $300 a month disability compensation from the Social Security Administration for being mentally ill. According to the New York *Daily News*, "A highly placed source within the Bureau of Disability Determinations [of the SSA] revealed that Berkowitz's eligibility is based on his inability to hold a job *because he is mentally ill* [emphasis added]."[15] Ideas, as Richard Weaver so aptly warned, have consequences.[16] (Actually, Berkowitz *is* holding a job: He is in charge of a special kitchen unit at the Attica prison.)

ACTING CRAZY AND BEING CRAZY

Berkowitz's new claims, as well as his initial claims, raise an obvious question: Was he pretending to be insane or was he really insane? The form of this question implies that *feigning insanity* and *being insane* are two distinct conditions. But that is not so. The appearance of this distinction is merely a consequence of our taking the medical metaphor of psychosis literally.

Feigning bleeding from a peptic ulcer and having a bleeding peptic ulcer are, indeed, two different conditions. But that is because the former consists of an act, of a pretense, of an impersonation of a person who bleeds from a peptic ulcer; whereas the latter constitutes a display of an objectively verifiable condition of the body, a bleeding ulceration of the stomach or duodenum.

However, as we have seen, "being insane" is an act, at least in the sense that it is an action rather than a happening. In Shakespeare's opinion, which I share, it is also an act in the sense that it is like a theatrical impersonation. But if being psychotic is like playing Hamlet, then feigning being psychotic is like feigning playing Hamlet, which would be the same as playing Hamlet. The point is that Hamlet is nothing but a role. No one *is*—or can *be*—Hamlet. An actor who plays Hamlet and an actor who impersonates an actor who plays Hamlet (there is a potentially infinite regress here) are both playing Hamlet, and are therefore indistinguishable from one another. Similarly, a person who "is" psychotic and another who merely "pretends" to be psychotic are both *acting* psychotic, and are therefore indistinguishable. (There may, of course, be different reasons why people act crazy, just as there may be different reasons why they play Hamlet; but these reasons or motives do not affect the *phenomenon* we see and observe, that is, "the psychosis.")

So whether Berkowitz was psychotic or was pretending to be psychotic comes down to the same thing: He was deceitful and dishonest. This was, indeed, clear in the quasi-theatrical dramatization of his madness, his claim that he is not David Berkowitz but the "Son of Sam." Obviously, this was a lie. Whether he was trying to deceive us, or himself, or both is something we cannot readily determine and may even be unknowable. Whatever the case, it has no bearing on the view I am presenting. Nor has the degree of deliberateness or "consciousness" with which Berkowitz was pretending any bearing on it. I am alluding here to some of my critics' attempts to rebut my argument by contending that Berkowitz (and others who act like he did) may not have been "fully conscious" of pretending to be the "Son of Sam"; that, perhaps, his imitation was "unconscious." But that is, again, beside the point: imitation is imitation, regardless of the actor's awareness of his behavior or his reasons for it.

Let us suppose, at least for the sake of advancing the argument, that behavior such as Berkowitz displayed by pretending to be the "Son of Sam" is deception. The fact remains—and it is a crucially important fact—that such a deception does not, by itself, constitute what we call a "psychosis." Actors, politicians, businesspeople, and many others engage in deceptions that do not, as a rule, lead to such a diagnosis. What is necessary to generate a diagnosis of psychosis is a certain kind of response in the audience—especially in authorities such as psychiatrists, lawyers, and judges—to the "patient's" deception. Such a response, defining the actor's performance in a particular way, results in a diagnosis of psychosis. And what is this required response? It is a psychiatric counter-deception, fitting and matching, like lock-and-key, the "patient's" deception. The "patient" asserts that he is not bad because the act was compelled by self-defense or by God or demons; the psychiatrist asserts that the patient is, indeed, not bad because the act was caused by his psychosis. The "patient" does not blame himself, and the psychiatrist does not blame the "patient." The crux of "psychosis" thus lies in a combination of such a reciprocal deception and counter-deception *together* with their official (medical, legal, and social) acceptance and accreditation as "disease" and "diagnosis." (This latter element is what has led some observers to speak of a "labeling theory" of psychosis [or mental illness].[17] Since everything in science, and indeed in everyday life, is "labeled" in one way or another, "labeling theory" is at once a poor term and a poor theory.)

The "Son of Sam" case illustrates very clearly this pattern of *deception* and *counter-deception* and their legitimization as *psychosis* and *psychodiagnosis*: David Berkowitz's *behavior*, consisting of an obviously staged caricature of a crazed maniac, was accepted as a "psychosis"; and the psychiatrists' *behavior*, consisting of an absurd caricature of a doctor examining a patient, was accepted as a "diagnostic determination."

What is always overlooked in this situation is that the psychiatrists—and the media and the public as well—had a choice: They could have formulated an altogether different view of these proceedings. As people regard a child impersonating a fireman as a childish game of "playing fireman," so they could have regarded Berkowitz's story about demons and dogs ordering him to kill as a grown-up game of "playing madman," and they could have regarded the psychiatrists' story about paranoia and psychosis as a grown-up game of "playing doctor." The point is: They didn't. Just as Berkowitz *chose* to kill and to act crazy, so the authorities *chose* to define him as psychotic. Now Berkowitz says that he is no longer interested in killing people, and some authorities say they are no longer interested in defining him as psychotic. But if Berkowitz was so "sick," how did he get "cured"? I raise that question here only to demonstrate how the idiocy of the belief that psychosis is a disease is matched by the idiocy of the belief that it can be "cured." (Of course, the "psychotic," like anyone else, can change his behavior. But abandoning a career of killing people is not a cure, just as embracing such a career is not a disease.)

THE PSYCHOTIC: SICK OR SICKENING?

The view that the term "psychosis" is typically used to characterize and condemn a particular action, rather than to identify a person's mental condition or the condition of the person's brain, is consistent with the fact that such a diagnosis is regularly made about *unknown* individuals. By "unknown individuals," I do not mean persons whom psychiatrists have not seen or examined. I mean individuals about whom nothing is known except that they have committed a particular act, and it is solely on the basis of that act that they are "diagnosed." For example, when President Kennedy was assassinated, the news media immediately characterized the unknown killer as "psychotic." People thus "knew" that the killer was crazy, even though they did not know who he was. A story in the *New York Times* in April 1980, headlined "Man Dies of Injury in Theater District," began with the following sentence: "A 26-year-old Baltimore man struck in the head a week ago by a chunk of plummeting debris near Times Square died Friday, and the police said yesterday they believed the incident and a similar one four days earlier were the work of a deranged rooftop assailant."[18]

Actually, what we are told about here is a person's behavior that is, both literally and figuratively, *sickening.* Whoever hurled these pieces of debris from New York rooftops (assuming the debris did not fall) made his victims sick, and indeed killed them. Furthermore, such a story is said to be "sickening" because hearing it makes us feel "sick." But notice the inexplicit and unacknowledged inversion of who is sick: not the victim, made sick by the injury; not those who read or hear the story; but the unknown perpetrator—who "must" be psychotic, for only psychotics do such things.

But if our idea of psychosis rests on the notion of acts that "only a psychotic would commit," then the concept of psychosis has clearly nothing to do with a "science" whose data are gathered by observing persons. Instead, the concept of psychosis constitutes both a cause and a consequence of a host of medical-ethical muddles and dilemmas, spanning a wide spectrum from homicide to suicide, from criminal insanity to civil commitability, from explaining behavior to excusing it.

What we can and cannot observe about so-called psychotic behavior, and what we do and do not know about the brains of persons who display such behavior, are clear enough. The claim that cerebral pathology or pathophysiology will one day be discovered in the heads of psychotic persons that will explain psychotic behavior is the ultimate in speciousness. Making such a claim is, in fact, simply advancing a presumption *as if* it were the most plausible of explanations. Asserting that a brain disease "causes" a person to engage in violent behavior and to offer certain kinds of justifications for it (such as then lead psychiatrists to diagnose a "psychosis") is like explaining and justifying behavior by attributing it to the will of God.

Finally, such a presumption brings us full circle back to the question of what should count as a disease: bad body parts ("lesions") or bad behavior ("bizarre violence")? If the former, then we must find the lesions before we can claim credit for them. If the latter, then we must distinguish those behaviors that we are prepared to accept as diseases from those that we are not (unless we wish to define all behaviors that displease us as diseases). The moral judgments and power relations that psychiatry has banished from its perception and conceptualization of psychosis thus return via the back door—leaving us with a concept that exemplifies the epistemological-ethical muddles of psychiatry itself.

NOTES TO CHAPTER 1

1. "Judge Orders Hospital to Free a Patient Held in Slaying of Husband," *The New York Times*, 1 August 1980, p. B-2.
2. *Ibid.*
3. See, generally, T.S. Szasz, *The Myth of Mental Illness* (New York: Harper & Row, 1961).
4. "6-year-old Killed in Hospital Rampage," *Syracuse Herald-Journal*, 24 June 1980, p. A-4.
5. V. Carriere, "Victim Got Killer Out of Hospital, Jury Told," *The Globe and Mail* (Toronto), 27 June 1980, p. 5.
6. *Ibid.*
7. " 'Son of Sam' Killer Berkowitz Says 'Urge to Kill,' Not Demons, Drove Him," *Washington Post*, 23 February 1979, p. A-3.
8. "Doctor Refutes Berkowitz," *Syracuse Herald-Journal*, 6 March 1979, p. 4.
9. B. Buyer, "Berkowitz Claims He Feigned Insanity to Justify Slayings," *Buffalo Evening News*, 1 August 1980, pp. 1, 4.
10. *Ibid.*
11. *Ibid.*
12. *Ibid*; see also B. Buyer, "Berkowitz Aiming to Block his 'Authorized' Biography," *Buffalo Evening News*, 2 August 1980, pp. A-1, A-12.
13. B. Buyer, "Claims for Disability Benefits Unauthorized, Berkowitz Says," *Buffalo Evening News*, 3 August 1980, pp. A-1, A-10.

14. R. Edmonds, "Son of Sam Taps Uncle Sam," *New York Daily News*, 5 June 1980, p. 4.

15. *Ibid.*

16. R. Weaver, *Ideas Have Consequences* (Chicago: Phoenix Books, 1962).

17. See, for example, T. Scheff, *Being Mentally Ill* (Chicago: Aldine, 1966).

18. R.D. McFadden, "Man Dies of Injury in Theater District," *The New York Times* 27 April 1980, p. 37.

2 THE CONCEPTS OF HEALTH AND DISEASE AND THEIR ETHICAL IMPLICATIONS

John Ladd

In this chapter, I propose to examine various conceptions of health and disease, relating them to the objectives of medical and health care and to general problems concerning the health of individuals and society. I shall argue that, for a number of reasons, certain prevailing concepts of health and disease are mistaken; and I shall offer as an alternative an analysis of these two concepts, the main thrust of which is that they belong to quite different categories and have quite different logical implications and practical consequences. There are, I shall argue, not only theoretical reasons for keeping these two concepts distinct, but also practical, perhaps moral, reasons for doing so. For, in my view, many of the serious ethical problems concerning health and disease that confront our society today can be traced to ideological and conceptual confusions concerning the nature of health and disease, and especially to the uncritical and generally unchallenged assimilation of the two concepts to each other, as opposite sides of the same coin. This conceptual assimilation leads inevitably to the identification of problems of health (which are essentially social problems) with problems of disease, namely, problems of treatment, cure, and prevention (which are essentially medical problems). Accordingly, the assimilation of the concepts of health and

A revised version of a lecture given to the Seminar in Bioethics, Fairfield University, May 6, 1980.

disease provides a theoretical background for what is often referred to as the *medicalization of American society*, that is, our society's penchant for treating social problems as medical problems and medical problems as social problems.

MEDICALIZATION AS A SOCIAL PHENOMENON

I shall begin with a few brief comments on "medicalization," as background for an understanding of the social implications of the analyses of the concepts of health and disease. What is meant by medicalization can be understood most easily by citing some well-known facts about the image of medicine and about what is called "health care" in America. First, the cost of so-called health care has skyrocketed—both for individuals and for society. It consumes an increasingly large proportion of the Gross National Product (GNP); by now, national resources devoted to health or medical care constitute almost one-tenth of the GNP. Nevertheless, it is commonly agreed that, proportional to the amount of dollars spent, there has not been a significant drop in mortality and morbidity rates.[1] Money is being poured down the drain, so to speak, and yet, perhaps partly for ideological reasons, our society is unprepared and unwilling to put the brakes on the cost of medicine.

Secondly, it is becoming increasingly obvious that our society, individually and collectively, is almost pathologically obsessed with health and medical problems. Our preoccupation with these problems can be observed almost everywhere: It is seen in television commercials and soap operas, in newspaper and magazine articles, in insurance advertising, in political speechmaking, in ordinary social conversation and in random gossip among friends, and in people's expressed personal concerns and worries. Indeed, Americans are often said to be a nation of hypochondriacs. It has even been alleged by some writers that the current explosion of interest in biomedical ethics provides additional evidence of the medicalization of our society. (To be fair, it should be observed that the same social phenomena have been reported in other Western countries.)

Thirdly, popular expectations about what medicine is able to do have risen beyond all reasonable bounds; at the same time, the scope of problems that are dumped in doctors' laps has also expanded. Physicians are regarded as the modern miracle-workers, who will soon discover the solutions to all our pressing problems, personal and social. As an indication of its supreme confidence (or overconfidence) in physicians and its enlarged demands on them, society has conferred extraordinary legal powers on the medical profession, which serve to promote and protect its monopolistic control over many facets of both our public and our private lives. Thus, by law and by convention, physicians exercise control over such diverse matters as the dispensation of drugs; pregnancy and childbirth; sexual activity; growing old; the treatment of the dying and the determination of death; access to and use of hospitals; health certification for jobs, for absence from work, for insurance, and for disability compensation; and so on.

These and similar trends show clearly that medicalization poses a challenge, if not a threat, to the well-being of our society. It has been described as "an insidious and often undramatic phenomenon accomplished by 'medicalizing' much of daily living, by making medicine and the labels 'healthy' and 'ill' relevant to an increasing part of human existence."[2] Ivan Illich is the best-known critic of medicalization; but we do not have to read his *Medical Nemesis* to know that our society has been medicalized as it never was before and to an extent that is rapidly approaching a crisis.[3]

Underlying medicalization in the sense intended here are two implicit propositions: the first is an "increasingly comprehensive idea of what constitutes health"[4] and the second is the assimilation of health care to medical care. The first of these propositions is epitomized in the World Health Organization's sweeping definition of health as "a state of complete physical, mental, and social well-being and not merely the absence of disease or infirmity." The second proposition implicitly assumed in medicalization is what has been aptly called "the great equation: Medical Care equals Health."[5] According to this equation, health is a medical concern, problems of health are medical problems, the objectives of health are medical objectives, and, in general, to care for health is to provide medical care. I shall argue that behind this equation of health care with medical care is the implied assumption that health is simply the absence of disease. This assumption will be examined later.

Putting these two propositions together, we can construct a syllogism that provides a certain rationale for medicalization. It runs as follows: If health is defined as "complete physical, mental, and social well-being," and health care is equated with medical care (i.e., the goal of medicine is assumed to be the "promotion, protection, and restoration of health"), then it follows that medical care, the doctor's job, is without limits and the scope of medicine extends to anything whatsoever that concerns an individual's well-being. The whole of life belongs to medicine.

On the other hand, if we balk at this surprising conclusion and hold instead that the province of medicine is essentially limited to the medical treatment that is provided by, say, physicians and hospitals, and that consists primarily of therapeutic measures such as the use of drugs and surgery, then we can keep the syllogism intact by simply circumscribing the notion of "complete well-being" and interpreting it as an entirely medical conception. Thus, given the two premises of the argument, we find ourselves logically forced to choose between accepting the unlimited scope of medicine or limiting our conception of human well-being to what can be taken care of by doctors. Medicalization as a social phenomenon seems to fluctuate between these two extremes, both of which promote the ascendancy of medicine. In fact, many people appear to believe in both sides of the dilemma simultaneously: They believe that all of their problems are medical and that doctors can take care of all of them.

It is hardly necessary to point out the absurdity of identifying well-being with health and of identifying health care with medical care. To begin with the latter, even if our medical resources were increased tenfold, our health problems still would not be solved, because according to the best estimates only 10 percent of our health needs (measured in terms of mortality and morbidity) are affected by the medical system.[6] Construed so narrowly, the pursuit of health (viz., well-being?) would appear to be a losing proposition. Someone might, of course, reply that we are now dealing with an altogether new concept of health, a scientific concept defined in medical terms (i.e., as the absence of disease). But that is to beg the question.

The equation of health care with medical care has so many ramifications that it would be tedious to dwell on them. It seems paradoxical to call a medical system designed to cope with disease a "health care" system, and insurance designed to pay the costs of medical treatment "health" insurance. Unfortunately, when we use such neologisms, we practice an insidious self-deception.

It is obvious that any serious critical discussion of medicalization (which, as I have pointed out, presumes the equation of health and medical care) must address the question: *what is health?* The rest of this essay will be principally concerned with some answers to this question. Perhaps the best way to begin is by examining the logical connections between the concepts of health and disease.

ARE HEALTH AND DISEASE CONCEPTUALLY INTERDEFINABLE?

In the literature on health and the health care system it is generally taken for granted that health and disease are interdefinable. Indeed, there is an almost universal assumption among medical and health care practitioners, among philosophers, and in the general public that health is equivalent to and may be defined as the absence of disease. It naturally follows from this assumption that if our aim is the promotion of health, then we should try to eradicate disease, an objective that might be said to be the aim of medicine.

Let us start with the question of interdefinability. Are the concepts of health and disease logical correlatives, that is, interdefinable in the same way as "dark" and "light," "odd" and "even," or "north" and "south"? If so, then "health" might simply mean the absence of disease or, conversely, "disease" might simply mean the absence of health. For example, to say that Smith is not healthy is to say that he has a disease and to say that he is healthy is to say that he does not have any disease.

Usually, when two concepts are found to be interdefinable, it is assumed that one of the pair is more basic than the other and that through the use of a definition the less basic concept can be eliminated and replaced by the more basic one. When used for purposes of elimination and replacement a definition is usually called a *reduction*. Definitions in general, and reductions in particular, may be introduced for clarification or to link the concept being defined to another set of concepts or to a theoretical framework.

As I have already indicated, "health" might be defined as the absence of disease or "disease" might be defined as the absence of health, depending on which of these terms is thought to be more basic for purposes of reduction. Those who choose to define "health" in terms of disease generally suppose that if "health" is defined in this way, it will be possible to clarify health issues by translating them into the more objective and scientific language of medicine.[7] On the other hand, those who choose to define "disease" in terms of health are generally interested in stressing the connections between problems of disease and wider social and value questions.

It should be easy to see the implications of adopting either of these reductionist definitions. Definitions of disease in terms of health tend to be expansive, general, and all-inclusive. The focus on health reflects the point of view of the layman and of society: They are concerned with disease only as it interferes with health. Humanistic and value concerns also loom large among those who adopt health as the basic concept. Definitions of health in terms of disease, on the other hand, tend to be restrictive, specific, and medical. By focusing on disease, the reductionist definition of "health" generally reflects the point of view of the professional medical practitioner, the scientist, and the technician.

Although philosophically unsophisticated discussions of health and disease usually do not reflect an awareness of the logical character of reductionist definitions—like M. Jourdain in Moliere's *Bourgeois Gentilhomme*, who suddenly learned that he had been talking prose all his life—it is easy for a philosopher to see that those who treat health in terms of disease and those who treat disease in terms of health are in fact speaking a reductionist language. Medicalization, as I have already observed, is based, either consciously or unconsciously, on a reductionist definition of "health" to disease; antimedicalism (e.g., the views of holistic health faddists) generally depends, consciously or unconsciously, on a reductionist definition of disease to health.

However, before committing ourselves to either one of these reductionist conceptions of health and disease, we must first ask whether the concepts themselves are in fact interdefinable. I shall argue that on closer examination we will find that the two concepts are not interdefinable, at least in the sense required for a reduction of one to the other.

The Case for the Incommensurability of Health and Disease

There are a number of arguments against the proposition that "health" and "disease" are interdefinable. A brief survey of them will help us understand some of the issues of concern here.

We might begin by noting that, etymologically, "health" and "disease" are unrelated. "Health" comes from an old English word whose cognates are "hale," "whole," and "holy." (And, of course, "healing.") We say that something is wholesome, meaning that it is conducive to health.[8] "Disease," on the other hand, comes from old French and incorporates the Latin prefix "dis," as it occurs in "disorder," "disarray," and so forth. As Dubos and others have pointed out, Greek mythology represents the two concepts by quite different personages: Hygeia and Asclepius.[9] There are also significant grammatical differences between the two words. "Health," in its ordinary usage, has no plural and, except in a manner of speaking, there are not different kinds of "health(s)." (The same grammatical peculiarity applies to "illness.") In contrast, the noun "disease" can be pluralized and there are many different kinds of diseases.

There are other significant differences between the two concepts. Health represents a general condition and, to a certain extent, an abiding condition; disease, on the other hand, reflects a specific, episodic, and often acute condition. Furthermore, "health" is also used not only specifically for good health, but also generically for a person's general bodily condition, as in one's "state of health," which may be good or bad. In this regard, "health" resembles grammatically some other generic words, like "intelligence"; such words are used to stand for both the general category and the preferred condition under that category. One is healthy when one's health is good and unhealthy when one's health is bad, just as one is intelligent when one's intelligence is high and unintelligent when one's intelligence is low.

This last consideration brings out another important difference between the concepts of health and disease. Health is a condition that allows of degrees; that is, a person can be in better or worse health,[10] one person can be healthier than another, and a person can be healthier at one time than at another time. Health embodies, as it were, a continuum of comparative degrees. Disease, on the other hand, does not allow of degrees or comparatives; one either has a disease or does not. That is not to say, of course, that a disease may not vary in severity, distress, development, or be in remission; but one cannot have more or less of a disease. It may be better to have one disease rather than another, but better or worse cannot be predicated of the disease itself.[11]

Being Healthy Versus Being Disease-Free

Perhaps the crucial difference between health and disease is categorical, for health is a dispositional property (capacity or power), whereas disease is an actual occurrent property. Thus, being healthy means more than simply not having a disease; at the very least, being healthy means, in addition, being *predisposed* not to have diseases. It is like an ability, the ability to cast off and recover from diseases. To say that a person is healthy implies a subjunctive or counterfactual conditional of the type that asserts that if the person in question is exposed to health hazards, invasive organisms, or traumas, that person will be less likely than others to contract a disease.[12]

The category difference between health and the absence of disease may be compared to the difference between "being safe" and "not having accidents." The safety of a building or of a driver consists of more than simply not having or having had any accidents; it entails that the thing in question has certain properties that render it unlikely to have accidents in the future and under a variety of different circumstances. To be safe means that if certain events were to occur, the thing in question would still be accident-free. Furthermore, the mere having of an accident does not necessarily prove that a building or driver was unsafe. The accident might be a freak. The not having of an accident is neither necessary nor sufficient to qualify a thing as safe.

Similarly, when we speak of a person as being healthy we mean that the person has the ability or the power (or strength) to resist diseases and to overcome them easily and quickly when assailed by them.[13] When one's body is under stress, it will quickly return to normal if one is healthy. To be healthy is not only to be free from actual disease, but also free from possible diseases or, to be more exact, comparatively free from them. Healthy people are much less likely than unhealthy people to succumb to diseases in general.[14] Health, in this sense, is connected with the notion of immune responses. I shall return to the notion of health as a capacity later.

Furthermore, health is something general that is predicated on a person as a whole. When we say that Mr. Jones is healthy, we are not saying that a particular part of him is healthy; it would be absurd to ask where he is healthy, although it is not at all absurd to ask where a person's disease is.[15] In general, then, "health" is used to refer to the overall condition of the organism rather than to the condition of a specific part of it. (Insofar as a particular organ is diseased, we might, of course, say that a person is ill or unhealthy on that account. But it usually does not follow that a person with a disease is therefore unhealthy; for example, if someone has athlete's foot or even a cold, it does not follow that the person is unhealthy.) Moreover, we do not ordinarily say that a person is unhealthy simply because of a particular disability or impairment; for example, a person may be completely healthy even though blind or an amputee. The important thing is the individual's overall capacity to resist diseases in general.

All these considerations suggest that when we speak of health we are dealing with a concept belonging to a different category from the category to which the concept of disease belongs. If this is so, then it follows that the concepts are not interdefinable and that it is not logically possible in any simple way to define "health" as the "absence of disease" or "disease" as the "absence of health." The concept of health, as I have argued, means something more than the mere absence of disease; perhaps, indeed, "disease" means something more than the absence of health.[16] So far, however, we have examined only the "logical" differences between the concepts of health and disease. We must now examine some of the positive ways in which health differs from disease.

POSITIVE THEORIES OF HEALTH

There are a number of positive theories of health; most of them are very general and, like the World Health Organization definition already cited, they are vague, and not particularly helpful for an understanding of the concept of health. Among such vague definitions are metaphysical conceptions of health that are presented in a specialized framework, such as definitions of health in terms of teleological wholeness or the harmonious ordering of bodily parts and functions.

In addition to freedom from disease and the capacity to resist disease, there are two other elements in the concept of health that should be mentioned. The first is the subjective aspect of health, namely, "feeling well" and "feeling fit." The second is the capacity to carry on various activities: If one is unhealthy, one cannot swim or play tennis, one cannot work, and one cannot fulfill many of one's responsibilities. Being in constant discomfort or having a chronic pain such as arthritis or migrane headaches combine these two aspects, for these "subjective" states generally incapacitate a person's daily activities.

The activity aspect of health is reflected in Talcott Parsons's oft-quoted definition of "health" as "the state of optimum *capacity* of an individual for the effective performance of the roles and tasks for which he has been socialized."[17] It should be observed that Parsons's definition of "health" relates it specifically to the individual's participation and status in the social system. Thus, his is essentially a sociological definition for use in describing and explaining certain kinds of social behavior. Although it does have the merit of calling our attention to the social component in the concept of health, this kind of definition is much too narrow for our purposes.

Three points must be noted regarding sociological definitions like Parsons's. First, such definitions do not make direct reference either to the subjective, affective side of health or to its physiological side. In particular, they do not refer to disease or other physiological or medical notions as components in the concept of health; although the latter are not part of the definition, we can assume that the definition allows for physiological causes and conditions of health and unhealth (sickness) insofar as they affect one's ability or inability to perform one's role and tasks.[18] In any case, Parsons's definition is not a reductive definition of the type criticized earlier, for it construes health as more than the absence of disease and positively affirms its social character.

The second point is that Parsons's sociological definition is too narrow, for it fails to incorporate references to other social facets of the concept of health besides roles and tasks. A wider social definition of "health" must refer to values. From that point of view, health is always something valued, just as unhealth or ill health, including illness and sickness, are disvalued. Broadly speaking, social conceptions of health accentuate the value side of health by relating it not only to roles and tasks, but also to wants, needs, expectations, social norms, and even to religious and magical beliefs and practices. Parsons's sociological concept of health fails to take into account these other value considerations.

The third point to be noted with regard to Parsons's definition and social definitions of "health" in general is that they have a built-in relativity, which, depending on one's anthropological positions regarding roles, values, societies, and cultures, may connect a wide range of capacities with being healthy or unhealthy. For example, in certain societies being fat is regarded as desirable, and in others, not; what to us appear to be abnormalities may seem perfectly normal or even desirable to persons in other societies. Myopia may be a distinct disadvantage for an individual living in a hunting society, whereas with glasses, it is not a disadvantage to someone in an industrial society. On the other hand, feeble-mindedness, as in Down's syndrome, is a distinct disadvantage in our society while it often is not in other societies. The list of such cultural differences is obviously very large. Parsons, it should be noted, allows for both universal and particular aspects of the roles and tasks that are used to define "health"; his definition avoids extreme relativism.

Nevertheless, it is important to avoid the pitfalls of relativism; in particular, what might be called "pernicious relativism," the view that matters of health are *completely* subjective and culturally determined. Pernicious relativism rules out any intersubjective or cross-cultural critique of health conceptions, for it follows from its basic assumption that it is impossible for societies (or perhaps even individuals) to be mistaken about their conceptions of health. Consequently, if such relativism is accepted, it would be [logically] absurd to engage in intersubjective or cross-cultural disputes about health. Like tastes, there can be no disputing matters of health and disease. But such a view is clearly untenable, for disputes about health are not absurd, as are disputes about taste; for one thing, they are more important, and for another, we can, do, and must engage in critical evaluation of health practices, in rational inquiry into health problems, and in rational argumentation about health matters.

A certain kind of relativism, which seems inevitable for the concept of health, need not be pernicious in the sense mentioned. Aristotle gave us a famous example of what might be called "rational relativism" by citing the case of the wrestler Milo, who is reputed to have eaten ten steer a day: What might be a small amount for Milo to eat might be a lot for a man who had just begun his training.[19] There is nothing irrational in saying that what is healthy for one person (or in one society) may not be healthy for another person (or in another society)—and the statement may be perfectly objective and even scientific.[20]

It does not follow that we must eschew every kind of relativism in order to be objective or even scientific about health. It would make things easier, however, if we used the term "contextualism" for the kind of relativism that is concerned with the dependence of the concept of health on particularities of age, sex, station in life, society, and culture. Not only are the conditions favoring health dependent on these factors; the content of the concept itself is also dependent. By virtue of its contextualistic character, it follows that there is no single paradigm of health that applies to everyone regardless of age, sex, culture, and so forth.

HEALTH AND ADAPTATION

As I have suggested, a sociological definition of "health" like Parsons's is excessively narrow.[21] Let us therefore turn to a contextualistic theory, namely, a theory put forward by René Dubos defining health in terms of adaptation to the environment. Although the concept of adaptation is very general and vague, it can be specified in a number of directions by detailing the challenges arising in different sorts of environments as well as the support these environments offer: internal and external, physical and social. In his *Mirage of Health*, Dubos describes in some detail how this adaptation takes place and how the various responses to the challenges of the environment are developed.

Dubos's book brings out several significant features of the concept of health. First, health is not a unitary concept; it does not represent a uniform, Platonic ideal that all human beings and all human societies should strive for. Rather, "health" must be contextually defined: that is, to determine what health is we must determine what is healthy for X in situation Y under circumstances Z. The case of immunity against infectious diseases provides a good illustration of the contextual character of health: being a carrier of the sickle cell anemia gene (a heterozygote) confers a degree of immunity against malaria; hence, in former times, people living in tropical Africa who were sickle cell carriers where malaria was rampant were "healthier" than the rest of the population because they were resistant to malaria. On the other hand, their descendants in the United States do not need to be protected against malaria, and because of other undesirable aspects of being a sickle cell carrier, those who are carriers may be said, *pro tanto*, to be less healthy than those who are not.

GENERAL REMARKS ON THE CONCEPT OF HEALTH

In order to elucidate the general features of the contextualistic concept of health that I have in mind, it may be worthwhile to contrast the positive concept of health with a positive concept of disease. Since it is not possible to undertake an analysis of the concept of disease here, I shall merely make a few remarks about it.

Disease, in the sense that concerns us here, is basically a physiological concept. Thus, in *Stedman's Dictionary* we find disease defined as "an interruption, cessation or disorder of body functions, systems or organs."[22] Likewise, *The Shorter Oxford English Dictionary* defines disease (definition 2) as "A condition of the body, or of some part or organ of the body, in which its functions are disturbed or deranged."[23] We may also take note of Henrik Wulff's definition of a "disease entity" as "the vehicle of clinical knowledge and experience."[24] I shall treat the abstract term "disease" as the name of the class of specific diseases of the sort used in disease classification and diagnosis. There are many ways of classifying diseases, but the general purpose of using a "disease entity" in a particular diagnosis is to connect signs and symptoms (manifestations) with a prognosis and with a determination of how the disease in question will be affected by different sorts of treatment.

If we put together all these points, the concept of disease will emerge as a very specific concept, ordinarily referring to something locatable in some place in the body, and characteristically clinically oriented; in other words, the concept of disease is primarily a technical medical concept. As such, it may be said to be a *closed* concept as compared with the concept of health, which, if we accept the analysis presented here, is an open concept. It is unnecessary to specify in any more detail the senses in which the concept of disease is closed. Suffice it to say that disease is basically a clinical concept and, as such, it is conceptually linked to medical treatment in one way or another.

The concept of health, on the other hand, is *open* in a number of different ways. To begin with, it is multidimensional and involves a cluster of features. As a value concept, it is "open-textured," that is, the connection between its value aspects and various defining components in the concept is open—"fuzzy" to use Wittgenstein's term.[25]

INFLUENCES ON HEALTH VERSUS
CAUSES OF DISEASE

The conceptual difference between health and disease may be clarified by another distinction, namely, the distinction between influences on health and causes of disease. For influences on health, let
us begin by citing the four different "fields of health" that are used
by Lalonde to categorize the health problems of Canadians.[26] The
four fields are: (1) *Human biology*: genetic inheritance, the processes
of maturation and aging, and other things connected with the body
as a complicated biological organism; (2) *Environment*: things external to the body over which the individual has little or no control,
such as foods, drugs, air, water, and noise; (3) *Life-style*: matters
affecting an individual's health that are controlled by the individual's
decisions and habits; and (4) *The Health Care Organization*: resources
available through medical practice, hospitals, and so forth. The first
three fields are more important for our purposes than the last one. It
should be noted in passing that Lalonde's list places what I have
called "medical care" in the fourth and final category.

I use the term "influences on health" to refer to etiological factors in these three fields that contribute to health. Thus, "good
stock," genetically speaking, tends to endow a person with a natural
ability to resist and to overcome disease. A good environment also
contributes to a healthy society (people with the ability to resist and
overcome disease). Finally, a healthy life-style and healthy habits
tend to make healthy people.

The term "influence" is used because no single one of these factors is necessary or sufficient to make a person (or a society) healthy.
Each of these factors interacts with other factors and with unfore-
seeable circumstances to determine the outcome in particular cases.
The term "influence" is used to suggest that we are dealing here with
fuzzy concepts and open-ended categories.

What I have called "influences on health" may be contrasted with
the causes of disease. The most typical causal analysis of a disease
focuses on a necessary condition of the disease (e.g., a lesion or an
infectious agent), such that, if that condition is removed, the disease
in question will be cured or prevented. Thus, tuberculosis (TB) is
caused by the presence of tubercle bacillus in the sense that the presence of the bacillus is a necessary condition of having TB; it follows

that, in the absence of the bacillus in one's body, one cannot have TB. That is not to say, of course, that the presence of the bacillus in one's body is sufficient to cause the disease; there are a number of other conditions that favor or mitigate against having the disease. But for medical purposes, a necessary condition is all that is required.[27]

Not all clinical diagnoses and causal analyses are as simple conceptually as infectious diseases, but I submit that the objective of medical intervention, that is, treatment, whether it be preventive or curative, presupposes a fairly simple kind of causal analysis like the one just mentioned.[28] This side of clinical medicine explains both the stunning successes of modern medicine and its disappointing failures; for it fails when it is unable to identify the necessary condition of a disease, such as the cause of certain kinds of cancer.[29]

It is easy to see that the relationship between health and disease and the other factors affecting them, such as the contribution of the environment or of life-style, is not so easy to determine. We often know, as from epidemiological studies, that there is a relationship of some kind, but that is all we know for sure. For the most part, it is impossible to use this information in an individual diagnosis. Thus, it may not be amiss to call the relationships in question "open." Two examples will illustrate this point: the relevance of nutrition and of stress to health.

In *The Role of Medicine* Thomas McKeown argues persuasively that the extraordinary decline in mortality rates in the last two hundred years is due to improvements in nutrition rather than, as is commonly thought, to the development of hygienic measures related to such things as water supplies and sewage disposal.[30] He bases his conclusion on the fact that this decline in mortality rates antedates the introduction of hygienic measures and is correlated with an earlier improvement in food supply; there is further support for his conclusion in the fact that the decline in mortality rates reflects a decline in deaths from airborne infectious diseases, notably TB, rather than from waterborne or foodborne infectious diseases, which began to decline later. McKeown summarizes as follows:

> The appraisal of influences on health in the past suggests that we owe the improvement, not to what happens when we are ill, but to the fact that we do not so often become ill; and we remain well, not because of specific measures such as vaccination and immunization, but because we enjoy a higher standard of nutrition and live in a healthier environment. In at least one important respect, reproduction, we also behave more responsibly.[31]

The second example relates to stress. In a study of Boston middle-class families, Meyer and Haggerty observed that 21 percent of the children were positive for streptococci (from throat cultures), but only half of them had the associated clinical disease. They found that there was a definite association of both the acquisition of the streptococcus and the resulting illness with "chronic family stress." There have been many other studies that trace susceptibility to clinical disease to chronic stress in the family and on the job.[32]

There seems to be no doubt that both malnutrition and stress have an adverse influence on health, that is, the capacity to resist disease—especially in connection with infectious disease. My point is a simple one: *healthy people are less likely than unhealthy ones to get sick.* And the causes of good and ill health are largely social rather than medical. A brief list of the kind of conditions that make people unhealthy will suffice to show that the influences on health are largely social. Malnutrition (such as junk foods), smoking, obesity, and alcoholism account for most of our health problems as well as, directly and indirectly, for most of the unnecessary deaths and hospitalizations in our society. It is clear that medical intervention is not the solution to these problems; they are, rather, social problems.[33]

SOCIAL PROBLEMS VERSUS
MEDICAL PROBLEMS

The penchant for converting social problems into medical problems and for seeking medical solutions to these problems is pervasive in our society; I have referred to it as medicalization. It is, in a sense, a kind of escapism. We want quick and easy solutions: Technology is the model. For the most part, this kind of solution is what the medical establishment promises or, perhaps more accurately, is expected to deliver. In our society, we handle problems of stress by resorting to alcohol and drugs, and then we treat the resulting alcoholism and drug addiction as medical problems requiring medical treatment in pursuit of medical cures. By the same token, we handle teenage pregnancy, which is surely one of our most urgent social problems, by turning it into a medical problem and by trying to solve it through medical means (abortions) rather than addressing its basic social causes. We even consider hyperkinesis in children to be a medical problem rather than an educational or social problem.

There are many explanations for the use of medical solutions for social (and moral) problems. The social problems we face are most difficult and controversial; to solve them requires sacrifices of everyone, and at the same time requires a critical reexamination of the moral basis of our social life and of our favorite social institutions: the complex bureaucratic organizations dominated by mindless managers and vested interests. Instead of taking seriously our responsibilities for our health, as a society and as individuals, they are bypassed in the universal rat race for money, power, and prestige.[34]

NOTES TO CHAPTER 2

1. For facts and figures, see Herbert E. Klarman, "The Financing of Health Care," in John H. Knowles, ed., *Doing Better and Feeling Worse* (New York: Norton, 1977), pp. 215–34.
2. Irving Kenneth Zola, "Medicine as an Institution of Social Control," *Sociological Review* 20 (1972): 487–504. This article contains many penetrating observations on medicalization.
3. See Ivan Illich, *Medical Nemesis: The Expropriation of Health* (New York: Pantheon Books, 1976).
4. A good summary of the current state of medicalization is to be found in Renee C. Fox, "The Medicalization and Demedicalization of American Society," in Knowles, *Doing Better*, pp. 9–22.
5. See A. Wildavsky, "Doing Better and Feeling Worse," in Knowles, *Doing Better*, pp. 105–123.
6. Wildavsky, *Doing Better*, p. 105.
7. See, for example, Christopher Boorse, "Health as a Theoretical Concept," *Philosophy of Science* 44 (December 1977): 542–573.
8. For further details on the etymology of these terms, see *The Shorter Oxford English Dictionary* (Oxford: The Clarendon Press, 1964).
9. See René Dubos, *The Mirage of Health* (New York: Harper & Row, 1959), ch. 5.
10. Aristotle, "Health Admits of Degrees." *Nicomachean Ethics* 1173a24.
11. This is a logical point about the concept of disease, not a scientific one.
12. In this regard, being healthy is like being strong; a person can be strong even when not exhibiting his or her strength, and a strong person can be subdued by superior force.
13. "Health is a margin of tolerance for the inconstancies of the environment." Georges Canguilhem, *On the Normal and the Pathological*, trans. Carolyn R. Fawcett (Dordrecht, Holland: Reidel, 1978), p. 115.

14.   Epidemiological information about the spread of infectious diseases attests to the fact that healthy people are much less susceptible to them than others (e.g., TB). See Thomas McKeown, *The Role of Medicine* (London: Nuffield Trust, 1976).

15.   The same considerations hold for the words "ill" and "sick." I have not specifically discussed the terms "illness" and "sickness," which represent notions that share some of the category properties of both health and disease. However, in contrast to the latter, "illness" and "sickness" generally have subjective connotations; for example, one says: "I feel ill" or "I feel sick." I shall discuss these particular notions later.

16.   "Disease is a positive, innovative experience in the living being and not just a fact of decrease or increase. The content of the pathological state cannot be deduced, save for a difference in format, from the content of health; disease is not a variation on the dimension of health; it is a new dimension of life." Canguilhem, *On the Normal*, p. 108.

17.   E. Gartly Jaco, ed., *Patients, Physicians and Illness*, 3rd ed. (New York: The Free Press, 1979), p. 123.

18.   See Parsons's theory of the sick role.

19.   Aristotle, *Nicomachean Ethics* 1106b5.

20.   As Parsons points out, we should not tie the concept of health too closely to the idiosyncratic preferences and conduct of the individual concerned. Thus, a person can be perfectly healthy but not healthy enough to climb Mt. Everest or to be a deep sea diver. Very old people and infants may be perfectly healthy, but they cannot do everything that a person in the prime of life can; that is why Parsons ties the concept of health to social roles and social tasks.

21.   To be just to Parsons, we must remember that his purpose in defining health in sociological terms is sociological rather than ethical.

22.   *Stedman's Medical Dictionary* (Baltimore: Williams and Wilkins, 1976), p. 401.

23.   *The Shorter Oxford English Dictionary* (Oxford: Clarendon Press, 1964), vol. 1, p. 524.

24.   Henrik R. Wulff, *Rational Diagnosis and Treatment* (Oxford: Blackwell Scientific Publications, 1976), p. 66.

25.   See J.M. Brennan, *The Open-Texture of Moral Concepts* (New York: Barnes and Noble, 1977).

26.   Marc Lalonde, *A New Perspective on the Health of Canadians* (Ottawa: Information Canada, 1974).

27.   Obviously, this statement needs further qualification. The analysis of cause presents many complications, both on the philosophical and on the medical level.

28.   I do not want to say, of course, that medical diagnoses are themselves simple and straightforward. I merely want to emphasize that the logical

structure of the causal analyses they involve is simple, at least relatively so. See Wulff, *Rational Diagnosis*, pp. 51–56.

29. There are, of course, also cures that have been discovered experimentally, as in the development of new therapeutic drugs.

30. Thomas McKeown, *The Role of Medicine* (London: The Nuffield Provincial Hospital Trust, 1976), especially pp. 61–66.

31. *Ibid.*, p. 94.

32. For references, see George W. Brown, "Social Causes of Disease," in David Tuckett, ed., *An Introduction to Medical Sociology* (London: Tavistock Publications, 1976), especially pp. 296 ff.

33. For further information on these matters, see Department of Health, Education, and Welfare (DHEW), *Healthy People: The Surgeon General's Report on Health Promotion and Disease Prevention*, DHEW (PHS) Publication No. 79-550713 (Washington, D.C.: U.S. Government Printing Office, 1979).

34. After completing this essay, my attention was called to a very interesting article: Michael H. Kottow, "A Medical Definition of Disease," *Medical Hypotheses* 6 (1980): 209–213. Dr. Kottow approaches the subject of health and disease from a slightly different point of view from mine. He distinguishes what he calls "core disease," which is a verifiable self-conscious sensation of dysfunction, from what he calls "conditioned disease," which is based on a sociocultural consensus. The essay is an attempt to avoid the problem of relativism, which I also discuss here, by connecting subjectively felt dysfunction and distress with objectively verifiable medical conditions. Dr. Kottow's concern is with the undefined area between what I call health and what I call disease.

I want to take this opportunity to express my gratitude to my old friend and colleague Sidney Cobb, M.D., from whom I have learned all that I know about preventive medicine and public health. He was the first to instruct me in the profound differences between positive health and the mere absence of disease.

3 THE SUBORDINATION OF THE CLINIC

H. Tristram Engelhardt, Jr.

Disease explanations indicate to physicians and patients the nature of the problems they address. Accounts of diseases, however, have varied widely in the history of medicine. Disease entities have been construed in terms of the causes of diseases, in terms of clinical findings, in terms of underlying pathophysiological processes, or at times as self-subsistent entities. The choice among these various accounts has implications for how patients are regarded, how they are treated, and how their complaints are understood. They direct the therapeutic imperative of medical language.[1] For example, an account that portrays diseases essentially as pathoanatomical and pathophysiological changes may discount patient complaints that are not easily referable to such changes. On the other hand, clinical accounts of diseases that construe them primarily as recognizable constellations of patients' complaints and physicians' findings would not as easily sustain such a bias against patient complaints. The primary concern would be whether the patient's complaints were part of a known cluster of complaints and findings recognized by medicine and amenable to some form of treatment, if only palliative.

In the contrast between pathological and clinical understandings of disease, one can identify a source of the difficulties in the contemporary care of patients. The more the reality of diseases is identified with pathoanatomical and pathophysiological changes, the less seriously physicians will take patients' complaints that are not easily accountable in those terms. A line is quite naturally drawn between bona fide complaints, those complaints accountable in pathoanatomical and pathophysiological terms, and male fide complaints, those complaints not amenable to such explanations. As Horacio Fabrega has argued, the development of a scale of pathoanatomical and pathophysiological truth values for patient complaints is a mark of modern Western medicine.[2] To some extent, complaints that fail to be so accounted for can be redeemed if they fall within established psychiatric categories. Otherwise, they are explanatory orphans and their bearers are placed within the lists of the worried well. They may be seen as having vague, unaccountable complaints that do not fall strictly under the aegis of modern medicine.

The roots of this modern understanding of diseases and patient complaints can be disclosed in part by an examination of some of the changes in the understanding of disease between the eighteenth and nineteenth centuries. These changes laid the bases for modern scientific medicine. They offered increased explanatory power and reliability of therapeutic intervention. They were, however, made at a price. They suggested that the primary focus of medicine was upon lesions of organs and of tissues, not upon patient complaints and clinical findings. The shift was from the bedside to the laboratory. This scientific and technological change has had obvious social consequences, ranging from the ways medicine is practiced to the ways patient complaints are understood.

In this chapter I will indicate some of the roots and consequences of this shift by reviewing a segment of the recent history of medicine and outlining several changes in the concept of disease between the eighteenth and the nineteenth centuries. In this fashion I will provide suggestions concerning the interplay of medical explanations and the character of medical practice. I will not examine here the ways in which the very concept of the pathological presupposes value judgments.[3] Rather, I will indicate how judgments about the reality of diseases have implications for the ways in which patients and patients' complaints are regarded.

DISEASE ENTITIES

There is a long history of discussion in medicine concerning the status of disease concepts and disease entities. Traditionally, discussion has focused on whether disease findings form natural kinds or artificial clusters of findings fashioned on the basis of human purposes. A major portion of these discussions have concerned the description of diseases, nosography, and the classification of diseases, nosology. The debate whether disease entities are natural or artificial classifications has been characterized in the history of medicine somewhat deceptively as a debate between ontologists versus physiologists of disease.[4] The notion of ontological concepts of disease is heterogeneous in that it encompasses various diverse understandings of disease. Some of them have construed diseases as self-subsistent organisms, or organizations of pathological cells. Others have seen diseases more as natural clusters of clinical findings, or perhaps in some cases as clusters of pathophysiological or pathoanatomical findings. There is, thus, an ambiguity in the traditional category of ontological accounts that can obscure the contrast between clinically oriented and pathoanatomically oriented accounts of diseases.

Consider, for example, the contrast between Thomas Sydenham's clinical accounts of diseases and the cellular-pathological accounts proferred by Rudolf Virchow. Sydenham (1624–1689), the noted English physician and colleague of the philosopher-physician John Locke (1632–1704), developed an account of diseases that gave its major accent to accurate clinical descriptions. It is in fact in the work of Thomas Sydenham that one finds the classical account of the natural history of diseases, the notion that diseases ought to be appreciated as reliably recognizable clusters of clinical findings. The Preface to the third edition of his *Observationes Medicae circa morborum Acutorum historiam et curationem*[5] contains, for example, an argument that diseases can be reduced to definite and concrete species of findings:

> Nature in the production of disease is uniform and constant; so much so that for the same disease in different persons the *symptoms* are for the most part the same; and the self-same phenomena that you would observe in the sickness of a Socrates you would observe in the sickness of a simpleton. Just so the universal characters of a plant are extended to every individual of the species; and whoever (I speak in the way of illustration) should accurately describe the colour, the taste, the smell, the figure, etc., of one single violet, would find that his description held good, there or thereabouts, for all the violets of that particular species upon the face of the earth.[6]

Sydenham directs the reader to a world of patients' complaints and clinical findings. He is interested in physiological and pathoanatomical accounts only after the clinical reality has been established and insofar as it is likely to be useful in providing actual treatment and reliable prognosis. Anatomy, pathology, or physiology would not be for him basic sciences, but rather auxiliary sciences. They alone could not offer an account of diseases, nor could they be the central focus of medical attention. It is clear that for Sydenham *medicine begins and ends in the world of patient complaints and clinical descriptions.* This is not to deny that Sydenham had interest in the causes of diseases, or in the equivalent of pathophysiological accounts of his day. He held, for example, that "Every specific disease is a disorder that originates from this or that specific exaltation, or (changing the phrase) from the specification of some juice in the living body."[7] The point of departure was, however, a reliable disease history, an account of a cluster of disease phenomena occurring in a pattern over time.

This contrasts starkly with the approach of the mature Virchow. Rudolf Virchow (1821–1902), the father of cellular pathology, argued for a pathoanatomical ontology of disease. The reality of disease was to be disclosed through the description of cellular pathological changes. Clinical findings were the manifestation of these basic, hidden realities. It was the scientist, not the clinician, who saw the disease in itself. As Virchow argued in his *Hundert Jahre allegemeiner Pathologie*[8] " . . . here suffice it to say that, in my view, the disease entity is an altered body-part, or, expressed in first principles, an altered cell or aggregate of cells, whether tissue or organ. In this sense I am a thoroughgoing ontologist . . ."[9] In short, a disease is an aggregate of deranged cells.

The shift from clinically oriented appreciations of disease to a generally accepted pathoanatomical and pathophysiological account of disease was occasioned by complex forces. In part, they involved the rejection of the elaborate nosologies of the nineteenth century and the arbitrary character of many of their taxa. This rejection was widespread, variously expressed, and encouraged by the early nineteenth century successes of pathoanatomical investigations. The early Virchow, in contrast to the later Virchow, who found a place for ontological views in pathology, vehemently attacked the ontologists: "Ever since we recognized that diseases are neither self-subsistent, self-contained entities, nor autonomous organisms, nor entities that have invaded the body, nor parasites rooted in it, but rather that they represent only the course of corporeal appearances under changed conditions—since this time, healing has had to compass maintaining or restoring the normal conditions of life."[10] The young Virchow is, in short, rejecting every form of ontology, not just clinical ontologies of disease.

Similarly, the physiologist Carl Wunderlich (1815–1877) speaks to the inadequacy of ontological accounts because they lead to treating classificatory units as things, "Presupposing them as actually existing and at once considering and treating them as entities . . . [but] which contain no truly essential feature and to which we only, by way of accepting, or by using compulsion, find an example in nature."[11] In their rejection of ontological accounts of disease, Virchow and Wunderlich reflected F.J.V. Broussais's (1772–1838) classical criticism of ontological theories. Broussais particularly had in mind French nosographers such as Philippe Pinel (1745–1826): "One has filled the nosographical framework with groups of most arbitrarily formed symptoms . . . which do not represent the affections of different organs, that is, the real diseases. These groups of symptoms are derived from entities or abstract beings, which are most completely artificial ortoi; these entities are false, and the resulting treatise is ontological."[12] The descriptions which Sydenham had pursued in the hope of discovering true and reliable accounts of diseases were dismissed as failing to accord with reality.

One sees, in summary, a major shift in interest regarding nosography and nosology. Where many eighteenth century physicians were committed to developing ever more reliable descriptions of diseases and classifications of clinical findings, these nineteenth century physicians rejected them as generally useless elaborations of the human mind, bearing at best a distant connection to reality. Such a loss of confidence in the reliability of clinical descriptions in and of itself would have marked a radical change in the appreciation of clinical findings. It was, however, bound to a major development in medicine: successful pathoanatomical, pathophysiological, and bacteriological accounts of disease. These accounts revolutionized the understanding of medicine. They provided ways of recasting the old world of clinicians in terms of a new world of basic scientists. What had previously been unconnected signs and symptoms could now be understood and related in terms of an underlying account: for example, the appreciation of general paresis as a form of syphilis, or the development of the concept of the disease of tuberculosis, uniting the findings of scrofula, hemoptysis, consumption, and Pott's disease. On the other hand, diseases that had been confused came to be appreciated as separate disease entities: for instance, typhus and typhoid were confused as late as the end of the nineteenth century,[13] and the clinical category gonorrhea originally embraced not only the consequences of infection with Neisseria gonorrhea, but of chlamydiae and T. mycoplasma as well.[14] One might note that it was not until very recently that the last two were seen as causes for a great deal of what had been characterized in the past simply as non-specific urethritis. This distinction led to a further elaboration of disease entities.

Such developments of new descriptions and classifications of diseases came out of a commitment to pathoanatomical and pathophysiological, and later bacteriological, research. Although such research antedated the nineteenth century (for example, Giovanni Morgagni's 1761 *De sedibus et causis morborum per anatomen indagatis*[15]), it was not until the nineteenth century that it began to bear fruit generally. For example, one can sense the excitement of Xavier Bichat (1771–1802) when he was able to account for the pathoanatomical basis of jaundice. It is a change in viewpoint that marked the nineteenth century: "Jaundice has been for a long time considered by practitioners as an essential malady; post-mortem examinations have also proven that this affection, thought primitive, was in reality only consecutive to diverse alterations of the liver, of which it is always a symptom."[16] Through the development of a science of pathoanatomy, the focus of medicine went inside the body. What had been a maze of clinical findings was now to be successfully negotiated with the help of pathoanatomical studies, and later with the aid of physiology and bacteriology. The promise was immense and, as soon became apparent, well-founded. The confusion and interminable disputes about the causes and natures of diseases that had traditionally plagued medicine appeared now in principle to be open to resolution. The character of medicine changed, and a sense of major progress was instilled.

What began in the autopsy room and in the laboratories of the basic sciences came to flourish in the laboratories of hospitals. Twentieth century clinicians have brought the deliverances of nineteenth century laboratory medicine into the context of ordinary care. Clinicians who in the eighteenth century would have been forced to rely upon clinical findings to sort out the significance of an illness can now rely upon laboratory tests ranging from pathological determinations to the culturing of bacteria. The sense of what it means to identify a disease entity has changed.

These developments suggested that the *real* reality of medicine lies within. As Broussais put it, " . . . true medical observation is that of the organs and their modifiers, it is, in fact, an observation of the body itself . . ."[17] This point has been repeated again and again in the nineteenth and twentieth centuries. The traditional clinical pathological conference was a dramatization of this point. The internist was given the findings associated with the illness of a recently deceased patient. After the internist attempted correctly to diagnose the patient's disease, the pathologist gave the final and true account. To again underscore Horacio Fabrega's point: complaints became understood in terms of their pathophysiological truth values.[18] They could be understood and dealt with only insofar as they could be understood and dealt with by the basic sciences.

In other words, with the triumph of pathoanatomical studies, patients' complaints needed to be reunderstood, translated in terms of the pathoanatomical, and later pathophysiological and microbiological, nosologies of modern medicine. As traditional findings were cast into new nosological grids, the old descriptions themselves changed as the data were seen in new contexts. Fevers were no longer essential fevers, but fevers due, for example, to particular infections. The data were thus essentially altered. Fever was appreciated as a symptom, not as a disease. For instance, if one looks at William Cullen's (1710–1790) classification of fevers, one finds the category "synochus" described as "Contagious. A fever compounded of synocha and typhus; at first a synocha, afterwards and towards the end a typhus."[19] For Cullen, a synocha is a continuous fever characterized as "Heat much increased; pulse frequent, strong and hard; urine red; the functions of the sensorium but little impeded."[20] And typhus is described as: contagious; heat but little increased; pulse small, weak, generally quick; urine little changed; the functions of the sensorium much impeded; great prostration of strength.

> 1. Typhus *petechialis*; generally attended with petechiae.
>   This varies in degree.
>   a. T. mitior.
>   a. T. gravior.
> 2. Typhus *icterodes*; with yellowness of the skin.[21]

We array the data quite differently. On the one hand, we have come to quantitate fevers, an innovation of the late nineteenth century. (Although Hermann Boerhaave [1668–1738] used a thermometer, the originator of modern clinical thermometry was Carl Wunderlich.) Given our excellent qualitative data, we have ceased to be as attentive as our clinical forefathers were to the rhythm and qualities of fevers. On the other hand, and more importantly, we possess a different sense of what is relevant and useful.

The world of medicine appears differently to us than to our eighteenth century antecedents, even before we consciously interpret it differently. The theoretical presuppositions of the basic sciences have come to structure the everyday experience of illness by both physicians and patients. The world of the clinic has changed through a dialectic in which clinical findings have been reinterpreted in terms of the nosologies of the basic sciences, which have in turn delivered new clinical descriptions, which are themselves then submitted to further revision, given further changes in basic scientific appreciations of disease. The result is an interplay between clinical and pathological findings; this interplay now characterizes all mature branches of medicine. In fact, for us a mark of the immaturity of a field, such as psychiatry, lies in its incapacity to play off and test its clinical findings against pathoanatomical and pathophysiological findings. For most areas of medicine this heuristic dichotomy has been fashioned between what may be called illnesses, or more generally, to use Clouser, Culver, and Gert's term, "maladies"[22] on the one hand (i.e., first and third party complaints about being sick, disabled, deformed), and theoretical accounts of illnesses framed in pathoanatomical and pathophysiological terms on the other (these one might stipulatively call diseases).[23] Illnesses are then related, as far as possible, to the orthodox disease entities of the basic sciences. Clinical disease entities are seen as provisional, as constructs awaiting an account through the basic sciences.

THE SUBORDINATION OF THE CLINIC

Much of this major change from the world of the clinic to that of the laboratory has been sketched in Michel Foucault's *The Birth of the Clinic*.[24] Unfortunately, however, he fails to underscore two essential points. First, far from having chronicled the birth of the clinic, he has in fact given the story of its subordination to the laboratory. Though he depicts the advances of Bichat and Broussais, he fails to stress that these brought with them an ideology that led to discounting patient complaints that are not easily or readily explicable in pathoanatomical or pathophysiological terms. Secondly, he does not sufficiently acknowledge the empirical clinical concerns of clinicians such as Sydenham and his successors François Boissier de Sauvages (1707–1767) and William Cullen. It is almost as if in his portrayal of them as rationalists who would eschew, if possible, the distractions of actual patients,[25] he were seeing them not through their own works, but through the account of ontologists provided by Broussais.

The first failure prevents drawing an important moral on the basis of the comparison of a clinically based and what might be termed basic science-based medicine. A wholesome judgment would be that each offers only a partial account of medicine. On the one hand, the approach of the eighteenth century clinicians required taking the complaints of patients seriously. It is, after all, from the problems of patients and the problems of others with patients that medicine developed as a social enterprise. On the other hand, medicine needs reliable explanatory and predictive accounts. Insofar as they succeed, interest in them takes on a life of its own, apart from whatever original inspiration it might have had with respect to the actual care of patients and the prevention of illness. They are pursued as independent scientific undertakings. However, it is in terms of interests in the prevention, cure, and amelioration of illness that the basic sciences are basic *medical* sciences, that is, bound to the enterprise of medicine.

In this sense, what we call the basic sciences are irremediably auxiliary sciences with respect to medicine. They are fashioned so that patients can have their problems cared for. In other words, a distinction must be drawn between the basic sciences as very successful explanatory and predictive enterprise in their own right, and the basic sciences as auxiliary to the social goals and individual interests that direct medicine as an applied science. The point can be put in almost Hegelian terms. Both the clinical approach and the basic scientific approach are onesided and incomplete. Each requires the other. They are, if thus appreciated, a dialectical pair. Unfortunately, the understandable enthusiasm from the success of the basic sciences has often obscured this point and led falsely to considering as male fide those patient complaints unamenable to full explanations within the basic sciences.

This distrust of nonpathoanatomically or pathophysiologically based complaints has become integral to the character of modern Western medicine. One finds it in the ways medical students and interns refer to patients with recurring but nonspecific complaints as "crocks." Such patients fail to be assimilable within the scientific model, in terms of which the high technology hospitals associated with medical schools are organized. As a result, not only general or family practice, but much of primary care medicine appears puzzling to such physicians when they enter practice. It is rich with individuals presenting to physicians with vague complaints that cannot be easily referred to particular pathophysiological or pathoanatomical lesions. These patients come seeking care for complaints, as patients have come for millennia. Often, given the reigning model, they themselves may seek an account in terms of the basic sciences. In other circumstances, they may simply wish to have their complaints recognized and taken seriously.

The roots of this clinically oriented element of medicine can be appreciated if one turns to the contribution of the eighteenth century nosologists. Here Foucault's second failure strikes home. In his account of the birth of the clinic, he also failed to underscore the important and enduring contribution of the eighteenth century clinicians. The case of François Boissier de Sauvages (1707–1767) provides an excellent example. Because of the failure of theoretical accounts based on iatromechanical, iatrochemical, or other explanatory frameworks to provide successful explanations or guides for therapy, Sauvages followed Thomas Sydenham's Baconian faith in clinical description. He, as Sydenham, took botany as the exemplar science, as one can see from the title of his 1763 work, *Nosologia methodica systens morborum classes juxta Sudenhami mentem et botanicorum ordinem.*[26] Sauvages in addition had been in correspondence with Carl von Linnaeus,[27] and Linnaeus had published a clinically based nosology also in 1763, under the influence of Sauvages.[28]

Sauvages's world of diseases accents patients' problems and clinical findings. Given this approach, pain becomes a major and immediate focus of medical interest. The result is a quite different way of understanding the world of medicine. One can see this from Sauvages's catalogue of over 2,000 species of disease, which, in the

1768 edition of his *Nosologia methodica*, he placed under 317 genre and within 10 classes: defects or superficial affections (vitia seu affectus superficiarii), fevers (febres), inflammations (phlegmasiae), spasms (spasmi), problems with breathing (anhelationes), debilities (debilitates), pains (dolores), madnesses (vesaniae), fluxes (fluxus), and constitutional disorders or deformities (cachexiae; morbi cachectici seu deformitates).[29]

Because medical reality was not seen to be basically pathoanatomical or pathophysiological, patient complaints with or without such obvious bases were not discounted. Clinically recognized constellations of patient complaints could be acknowledged on their own merit. Though particular correlations of clinical findings with pathoanatomical findings were recognized and explored, a pathoanatomical underpinning was not necessary to authenticate a complaint. For example, in Sauvages one finds the nosological taxon *anxietas agonistica*, the anxiety of death or the dysphoria that accompanies the imminence of death.[30] It was not seen to have a specific pathological basis. It was still of special clinical concern. The problem was addressed even though the underlying derangements could not be. As anxieties are generally, it was seen to be a form of pain, of the order "vague or wandering pains that do not have a name from a fixed site" or "vague or wandering pains or vexations."[31] *The clinically problematic held central stage.*

The triumph of the basic sciences in the nineteenth century changed this. It introduced a diagnostic ideology that gave priority to that which could be referred to pathoanatomical lesions or pathophysiological disturbances. Even family physicians who invest a great proportion of their time in treating the problems of the worried well and vexed ill often conceive of their task as either making a pathoanatomically or pathophysiologically based diagnosis, or referring a patient to a specialist in order to establish such a diagnosis, or as deferring such a diagnosis until data are available to allow such a diagnosis. But such an attitude presumes that data that do not support a pathoanatomically or pathophysiologically based diagnosis, when they concern some variety of vague pains or vexations, cannot at times suffice in their own right. As a consequence, the American Academy of Family Practice has not followed the example of the American Psychiatric Association[32] and attempted to devise a diagnostic and statistical manual that will allow better discrimination of the kinds of problems often brought by patients to family physicians, such as the problems of the worried well and the vexed ill. There has not been a serious, major intellectual attempt to chart that territory in terms of possible diagnoses and treatments. Such an approach, however, would have found support within the undertakings of nosologists such as Sauvages. One would want to be able to discriminate as best as possible the ways in which people are worried well or vexed ill in order to develop better means of addressing their problems. Such an undertaking, however, would presume that clusters of patients' complaints could be foci of legitimate intellectual interest in medicine, even where attempts to disclose pathophysiological and pathoanatomical undertakings had failed. The fact that such undertakings are not pursued is an expression of the clinic's subordination to the laboratory.

Pathoanatomically or pathophysiologically based accounts of disease indicate which kinds of complaints are likely to be more easily accounted for and more easily treated. The focus of interest falls understandably on such problems and not on those that are resistant to generally successful explanatory models, and which, therefore, do not promise therapeutic success. Further, since medical schools and hospitals, where most residents are trained, tend to be high technology institutions, this bias will be strengthened. The most rewarding cases will be those from which one can learn more about the accepted explanatory models and the ways they can be successfully applied to the treatment of patients. Insofar as these models work, this will all be well and good. The difficulty is when these interests fail to be balanced with an appreciation that much of what patients want from medicine does not fall within the compass of high technology medicine. It is made worse when it is allowed to produce an ideology suggesting that the complaints not easily amenable to high technology medicine are not truly medical.

CONCLUSIONS

Patients and their problems are understood in terms of the goals of medicine. If these are construed primarily as understanding and treating pathoanatomical lesions and pathophysiological disturbances, complaints not grounded in particular lesions and disturbances will not be considered bona fide. Individuals who proffer such complaints in the attempt to be considered as patients will, in varying degrees, be appreciated as individuals acting in bad faith. They will be seen as attempting to misuse medicine and to distract it from its important central and serious missions in order to direct it instead to undertakings that properly fall outside its borders. If, however, medicine is understood as an attempt to address complaints that individuals bring for a variety of reasons, ranging from unwanted pains and physical and psychological dysfunctions to deformities and absences of physical grace, medicine will have a different cast. Granted, physicians will need to have boundary criteria so that they can, when it is important, distinguish medicine from undertakings in public order, education, and religion. That is, physicians will for the most part restrict themselves to complaints of a physical or psychological (as opposed to those of a religious or social) nature, held to be embedded in chains of physical and psychological causality beyond individuals' direct and immediate control. Because of the ambiguities, one "problem" is likely to be addressed by more than one profession. A problem with excessive drinking, for example, is likely to be claimed not only by medicine but by law, religion, and ethics as well. But the point here is that insofar as physicians would see it to be a problem amenable to their intervention, it is because, at least in part, they see alcoholism as embedded in psychological and physiological causal chains beyond the direct and immediate control of the individuals involved.[33] Thus, also, one finds William Cullen describing medical problems such as acute and chronic nostalgia.[34]

The moral is that physicians should not forget that medicine developed explanatory models in order to better treat patients' complaints. The former is secondary to the latter. Patients are interested in explanatory accounts, insofar as they are useful in solving their problems. However, given the scientific interests of physicians, especially academic physicians, whose rewards may not be in terms of resolving the problems of the worried well and the vexed ill, this may be obscured, if not forgotten.

NOTES TO CHAPTER 3

1. Christopher Boorse appears to miss the point about the therapeutic imperative of medical language. A patient visited with a diagnostic label is made a candidate for treatment. See "Health as a Theoretical Concept," *Philosophy of Science* 44 (December 1977): 542–573. William Goosens does

likewise. See "Values, Health, and Medicine," *Philosophy of Science* 47 (March 1980): 102; cf. H.T. Engelhardt, Jr., "Explanatory Models in Medicine: Facts, Theories, and Values," *Texas Reports on Biology and Medicine* 32 (Spring 1974): 225–239.

2. Horacio Fabrega, Jr., "Disease Viewed as a Symbolic Category," in H.T. Engelhardt, Jr., and S.F. Spicker, eds., *Mental Health: Philosophical Perspectives* (Boston: D. Reidel, 1978), pp. 79–107.

3. For a treatment of the points, see H.T. Engelhardt, Jr., "The Concepts of Health and Disease" in H.T. Engelhardt, Jr., and S.F. Spicker, eds., *Evaluation and Explanation in the Biomedical Sciences* (Boston: D. Reidel, 1975), pp. 125–141; and H.T. Engelhardt, Jr., "Ideology and Etiology," *The Journal of Medicine and Philosophy* 1 (September 1976): 256–268.

4. Peter Niebyl, "Sennert, Van Helmont, and Medical Ontology," *Bulletin of the History of Medicine* 45 (March 1971): 115–137; and Owsei Temkin, "The Scientific Approach to Disease: Specific Entity and Individual Sickness," in A.C. Crombie, ed., *Scientific Change* (London: Heinemann, 1961), pp. 629–647. For an interesting recent study, see F. Kräupl Taylor, *The Concepts of Illness, Disease and Morbus* (Cambridge, England: Cambridge University Press, 1979).

5. Thomas Sydenham, *Observationes medicae circa morborum acutorum historiam et curationem* (London: G. Kettilby, 1676). This work appeared in the first (1666) and second (1668) editions under the title *Methodus Curandi Febres, propriis observationibus superstructa*.

6. Thomas Sydenham, *The Works of Thomas Sydenham*, trans. R.G. Latham (London: Sydenham Society, 1848), vol. 1, p. 15.

7. *Ibid.*, p. 19.

8. Rudolf Virchow, *Hundert Jahre allgemeiner Pathologie* (Berlin: August Huschwald, 1895).

9. Rudolf Virchow, *Disease, Life and Man*, trans. Leland Rather (Stanford: Stanford University Press, 1958), p. 195.

10. Rudolf Virchow, "Über die Standpunkte in der wissenschaftlichen Medicin," *Archiv für pathologische Anatomie und Physiologie und für klinische Medicin* 1 (1847): 36, trans. S.G.M. Engelhardt in A. Caplan, H.T. Engelhardt, Jr., and J.J. McCartney, eds. *Concepts of Health and Disease* (Boston: Addison-Wesley, 1981), p. 188.

11. Carl Wunderlich, "Einleitung," *Archiv für physiologische Heilkunde* 1 (1842): ix (my translation).

12. F.J.V. Broussais, *Examen des doctrines medicales et des systemes de nosologie* (Paris: Mequignon-Marvis, 1824), vol. 2, p. 646.

13. William Stokes, *Lectures of Fever* (London: Longmans and Green, 1874).

14. In fact, gonorrhea meant "a dripping of seminal or pus-like fluid from the urethra or from the vagina." François Boissier de Sauvages, *Nosologia Methodica Sistens Morborum Classes Juxta Sydenhami Mentem et Botani-*

corum Ordinem, in 2 volumes (Amsterdam: Fratres de Tournes, 1768). Vol. 2, p. 277 (my translation).

15. Giovanni Morgagni, *De Sedibus et causis morborum per anatomen indagatis* (Venetiis: Ex Typographia Remondimiama, 1761).

16. Xavier Bichat, *Pathological Anatomy*, trans. Joseph Togno (Philadelphia: P. Grigg, 1827), p. 14.

17. F. J. V. Broussais, *De l'Irritation et de la Folie* (Paris: Delaunay, 1828); *On Irritation and Insanity*, trans. Thomas Cooper (Columbia, South Carolina; S. J. McMorris, 1831), p. ix.

18. Horacio Fabrega, Jr., "Disease as Symbolic Category."

19. William Cullen, *Nosologia Methodica*, trans. John Thomas (Edinburgh: J. Carfrae, 1820), pp. 121, 152.

20. *Ibid.*, p. 188.

21. *Ibid.*, p. 189.

22. K. Danner Clouser, Charles M. Culver, and Bernard Gert, "Malady: A New Treatment of Disease," *Hastings Center Report* 11 (June 1981): 29–37.

23. H. Tristram Engelhardt, Jr., "Clinical Judgment," *Metamedicine* 2 (October 1981): 301–317.

24. Michel Foucault, *Naissance de la Clinique* (Paris: Presses Universitaires de France, 1963); *The Birth of the Clinic*, trans. A. M. Sheridan Smith (New York: Pantheon Books, 1973).

25. "In the rational space of disease, doctors and patients do not occupy a place as of right; they are tolerated as disturbances that can hardly be avoided: the paradoxical role of medicine consists, above all, in neutralizing them, in maintaining the maximum difference between them, so that, in the void that appears between them, the ideal configuration of the disease becomes a concrete, free form, totalized at last in a motionless, simultaneous picture, lacking both density and secrecy, where recognition opens of itself onto the order of essences. Classificatory thought gives itself an essential space, which it proceeds to efface at each moment. Disease exists only in that space, since that space constitutes it as nature; and yet it always appears rather out of phase in relation to that space, because it is manifested in a real patient, beneath the observing eye of a forearmed doctor." Foucault, *The Birth of the Clinic*, p. 9.

26. François Boissier de Sauvages de la Croix, *Nosologia Methodica Sistens Morborum Classes Juxta Sydenhami Mentem et Botanicorum Ordinem*, in 5 volumes (Amsterdam: Fratres de Tournes, 1763).

27. Fredrik Berg, "Linne et Sauvages: Les rapports entre leurs systemes nosologique," *Lynchnos* (1956): 34.

28. Carolus Linnaeus, *Genera morborum in auditorum usum* (Upsaliae: Steinert, 1763).

29. Sauvages, *Nosologia Methodica* (1768), vol. 1, pp. 92–95, 100; vol. 2, p. 433.

30.   *Ibid.*, vol. 2, p. 38.

31.   *Ibid.*, cf. vol. 1, p. 94; vol. 2, pp. 1, 37–39.

32.   American Psychiatric Innovations, *Diagnostic and Statistical Manual of Mental Disorders*, 3rd ed. (Washington, D.C.: American Psychiatric Association, 1980).

33.   For a more detailed study of the problem of the boundaries of medicine, see H.T. Engelhardt, Jr., "Doctoring the Disease, Treating the Complaint, Helping the Patient: Some of the Works of Hygeia and Panacea," in H.T. Engelhardt, Jr., and D. Callahan, eds., *Knowing and Valuing* (Hastings-on-Hudson: The Hastings Center, 1980), pp. 225–249.

34.   William Cullen, *Nosologia Methodica*, pp. 121, 152.

4 TIME AND HEALTH CARE DELIVERY

Carl W. Nelson

"Here, on a bench a skeleton would writhe from,
Angry and sore, I wait to be admitted:
Wait till my heart is lead upon my stomach,
While at their ease two dressers do their chores."

> *In Hospital* "Waiting," William Ernest Henley

"Waste of time is thus the first and in principle the
deadliest of sins"

> *The Protestant Ethic and Spirit of Capitalism,*
> Max Weber

The contrast between institutional and patient "time" reveals value conflicts at the core of contemporary health care delivery systems. Although these value conflicts do not possess the sensational aura of other sociomedical-ethical dilemmas, they affect more people and highlight forces that underlie the health care delivery system itself.

I will argue that clock time in isolation presents an inadequate basis for examining temporal relationships in the delivery of medicine. Individual, or personalistic, time differs from institutional time. Moreover, individuals perceive the duration of time intervals differently from one another. Understanding the history, sources, and scope of these differences is a necessary first step toward their possible resolution.

It is immediately clear that clock time is important in the health services for technical and medical reasons. Prompt response to accidents and other acute conditions in emergency services, for example, often means the difference between life and death or serious functional impairment. Consider the massive training program of the citizens of Seattle, Washington in pulmonary resuscitation that has markedly decreased death rates from heart attacks.[1] The relationship between the spatial availability of emergency service and response time is obvious.

Once we move out of the technical domain, however, and into the subjective areas of psychological and behavioral factors associated with time perception and valuation, the effects upon health care behavior become more complex and contrast strongly with institutional clock time considerations. For example, we know that discrepancies between private time and clock time duration increase in altered states of consciousness, under stress, or under the influence of drugs or hypnosis. Mental depression and its negative views of the future constrict future time.[2] Chronically sick people, in general, are said to learn to reduce their desires, and their temporal horizons often become limited. Individuals who are forced to slow down their movements because of physical disabilities are often less aware of time dragging.[3] And, as will be discussed, age and socioeconomic and cultural factors also play an important role in influencing the perception of time duration, periodicity, and futurity.

The lack of individual control over time and events in institutional settings, where enforced idleness and anonymity and unclear or technically incomprehensible priorities prevail, also serves to further confuse and disturb individual conceptions of time. Most people, including physicians, are wholly ignorant of daily life within health institutions until they are forced to use their services. Isolation of the sick person from all but family and close friends in high technology institutions keeps us uninformed and unprepared for such experiences ourselves. When institutionalization occurs, regimented meal times, prescribed visiting hours, unexplained delays, and recurrent interruptions of sleep by staff or other patients can be both troublesome and debilitating. The two time systems, clock time for the institution forced to coordinate its resources and private time for the individual likely to be in a heightened emotional or drugged state producing new time perceptions, are clearly not congruent.

HISTORICAL CONSIDERATIONS

At one extreme, there is physical or clock time: unvarying and irreversible; equitably and unalterably distributed; not subject to accidents of birth, social systems, or chance; the time of science, economics, and institutions. Private time stands in opposition to physical time. It is personalistic and thereby influenced by events, perceptions, and values.

On the symbolic and semantic level, the evolution of the dichotomy between physical and personal time has a long history. For instance, we may consider the similarity between the Greek work for time, "chronos," and the Greek god, Cronus, who devoured his children.[4] Cronus was a child of Gaia (mother earth) and Uranos (father heaven)—thereby implying the early importance of the relative position of the earth and heavenly bodies in determining physical or clock time. But Cronus not only ultimately devoured his children, he first separated heaven from earth by castrating his father. By making ethereal or subjective time detached and impotent, while rooting physical time in worldly matters, Greek mythology also may have served to downplay psychological and personalistic time interpretations in favor of a more uniform and operations conception.

This view is compatible with Foucoult's study of the evolution of medical perception arising in the last years of the eighteenth century French "clinic."[5] He suggests that the patient had to be "enveloped in a collective, homogeneous, space." I would argue that temporal homogeneity is but another aspect of the drive to a common medical "perception" in clinical medicine and the teaching hospital. Foucoult writes:

> the clinic appears—in terms of the doctor's experience—as a new outline of the perceptible and statable: a new distribution of the discrete elements of corporal space (for example, the isolation of *tissue*—a functional, two-dimensional area—in contrast with the functioning mass of the organ, constituting the paradox of an 'internal surface') a reorganization of the elements that make up the pathological phenomenon (a grammar of signs has replaced a botany of symptoms), *a definition of the linear series of morbid events* [emphasis mine] (as opposed to the table of nosological species), a welding of the disease onto the organism (the disappearance of the general morbid entities that grouped symptoms together in a single logical figure, and their replace-

ment by a local status that situates the being of the disease with its causes and effects in a three-dimensional space). The appearance of the clinic as a historical fact must be identified with the system of these reorganizations. This new structure is indicated—but not of course exhausted—by the minute but decisive change, whereby the question: 'What is the matter with you?', with which the eighteenth-century dialogue between doctor and patient began (a dialogue possessing its own grammer and style), was replaced by that other question: 'Where does it hurt?', in which we recognize the operation of the clinic and the principle of its entire discourse.[6]

The scientific (and administrative) reorganization of Paris hospitals that Foucault analyzes was made necessary by the tremendous influx of population from the countryside, drawn by the promise of employment in the new factories of the industrial revolution. Hospitals themselves became the factories of the new medicine in which patients, physicians, and staff submitted (by different degrees) to the new discipline of clock time. The new wage system and emerging Protestant ethic in the period Foucault describes further objectified time by linking it to money. By the end of the nineteenth century, there were few family doctors who followed the old practice of never writing a bill, but of accepting what families could send, or considered a fair payment, usually around Christmas.[7] Payment was linked to the complexity and resultant time of service and was usually payable upon delivery. Fee-for-service physicians began to base and value their actions upon opportunity cost concepts by asking what alternative activities they could be performing in the same amount of time that would enable them to achieve their own goals of prestige, power, and financial strength. The sick patient, in contrast, had fewer opportunities to choose from in a world of limited medical resources, and was required to submit to prevailing rules and priorities. The discipline of urban factory life had prepared the patient to accept the subjegation of one's own time system for the time of the institution.

Since the industrial revolution, time and its passage has rarely been viewed in relation to *cyclical* events connected with *natural* phenomenon, such as growing seasons, tides, and astronomical events, but has become linked to *mechanistic* processes that are unvarying and irreversible.[8] Significantly, only medicine retains a leading role as mediator in the process of individual, irreversible, biological, and chemical change. Patients' faith in medicine's ability to forestall illness and decay, and in essence, to "conquer" time, leads them to willingly accept the perception, the temporal routine, and the control of the physician and hospital.

As this faith diminishes, or as alternative means of care become available, implicit value conflicts between patients and organized medicine become evident. Temporal value conflicts are among the most easily discernable conflicts that occur across a broad spectrum of health care activities. Although they will never capture newspaper headlines or result in court cases, these conflicts can tell us a great deal about what we value in medicine, how it is organized, and where it is heading.

SCHEDULING DECISIONS

Today the dominance of institutional time over personal time preferences is exacerbated in areas where medical resources are in short supply, poorly managed, or inequitably distributed. Kidney dialysis, surgical scheduling, and preventive services are three examples that illustrate the importance of these contributing factors. In each instance, patients' temporal preferences are often totally ignored, even where there is medical (as well as ethical) evidence to suggest that they should be given more consideration.

Kidney Dialysis. Since the Federal government's decision in 1972 to pay the costs of medical care for patients with kidney failure, the number of dialysis patients has increased more than ten times to approximately 70,000 people, and expenditures run over one billion dollars each year.[9] Patients must currently submit to a regimen of three four-hour to six-hour treatments per week, usually by visiting a dialysis center, where they are attached to hemodialysis machines by a permanent, surgically-created internal fistula so that blood waste products and excess fluids may be removed.[10]

Although facility dialysis nephrologists and personnel normally inquire about patients' preferences for dialysis scheduling times, high equipment utilization during day and evening hours is an important operating goal of each center. Because of limited resources, many patients will not be able to receive their preferred appointment times and must adjust their activities accordingly. Patients are often depressed, and nearly all have sexual problems and frequent medical complications. Opportunities for work, sleep, recreation, and the like are often limited. Life on dialysis, though it may be the only life available, is far from pleasant.

Critics have suggested that dialysis centers not only set operating hours for the convenience of medical personnel and schedules for maximum equipment utilization, but that many centers train a disproportionately low percentage of their patients for home dialysis. Proprietary kidney dialysis centers, such as those owned by National Medical Care, which control more than one-quarter of the market and are a virtual monopoly in some geographic areas, bear the brunt of much of this criticism.[11] Although some nonprofit centers train as much as 80 percent of their patients for home dialysis, proprietary centers average less than 10 percent. Since Medicare pays close to $30,000 a year for facility dialysis and approximately $15,000 for home dialysis, considerable financial interests are at stake. European countries, by way of contrast, have a two to three times greater proportion of patients who receive home dialysis.

Impressions that the quality of life is better for home dialyzed patients are hard to validate because of the lack of good objective measures and wide patient differences. However, it is undeniable that home dialysis offers more potential flexibility in scheduling treatments than facility dialysis. Controlling one's own treatment regimen, in one's own space, at times convenient to the individual and family members, is clearly desirable for a broad cross section of dialysis patients. In general, adjustment and rehabilitation of patients with chronic diseases is improved by giving them a full explanation of their disease and its treatment and as much responsibility as they can accept.

The one disadvantage of home dialysis from a temporal viewpoint is that it requires continual monitoring and assistance by a trained family member, friend, or paid technician. Monitoring and assistance in the patient's home is necessary because of the chance of equipment malfunction and the critical nature of the procedure as it is applied to chronically ill patients. Training can typically last eight weeks during the patient's regularly scheduled dialysis treatments at a facility dialysis center. Additional time needs to be spent in daily cleaning of equipment, changing the membranes that act as the artificial kidneys, and in doing paperwork associated with receiving reimbursable medical services. Many patients simply may not have family capable of tackling these considerable burdens and the psychological factors associated with life and death responsibility.

From the perspective of this chapter, the choice between institutional or home dialysis has distinct time implications. Home dialysis increases individuals' control of the occurrence, duration, and frequency of events that are no longer technically incomprehensible. Rather than locking patients into an immutable schedule, home dialysis enables patients to choose treatment periods that are flexible and that meet their preferences and those of their families.

Finally, a discussion of kidney dialysis is incomplete without considering a method that has begun to free many patients from institutional dependence without transferring the burden to one's family. This new alternative, Continuous Ambulatory Peritoneal Dialysis, involves putting sterile dialyzing solution *inside* the body, via a catheter implanted through the wall of the abdomen into the peritoneal (or abdominal) cavity. The peritoneum operates as the dialyzing membrane, and wastes pass across it into the solution filling the cavity. Every four to six hours during the daytime, and eight hours at night, the patient discards a plastic bag containing the toxin-bearing dialyzing solution before attaching a new container of sterile dialyzing solution to the catheter. Each exchange may take 30 to 45 minutes to perform.

There are, however, both medical and temporal psychological factors that may inhibit the adoption of machine-free peritoneal dialysis. Peritonitis, or inflammation of the peritoneum, remains a problem for patients following this technique. Users must be meticulous, trainable, and able to carefully perform the kinds of procedures that are vital to avoid contamination. Moreover, there is concern that patients subjected to seven-days-a-week treatment schedules that permit no intervals in which to escape their disease may be adversely psychologically effected. Some patients may simply prefer intermittent facility to home dialysis to avoid continuous and personal involvement in their own treatment. As of now we have no realiable method for determining who these patients may be and whether their preferences are immutable.

The issue of time in kidney dialysis is therefore one in which values will differ and conflicts are likely to occur. Patients indirectly compete against one another for preferred dialysis times on limited facility-owned equipment. Physician, staff, and institutional preferences for daylight work hours conflicts with many patients' preferences for nighttime dialysis in order to have uninterrupted hours for jobs or school. Home dialysis may cause conflicts due to the increased burden of assistance required by family members who have to give up their own time on a regular basis for the patient. Even continuous ambulatory peritoneal dialysis has a potential for individual internal value conflicts over time devoted to attending to one's own treatment and therefore made unavailable for other personal activities.

In kidney dialysis, as in other areas where alternative treatment methods are available, an appropriate ethical position should incorporate the principle of informed choice. In addition to presenting patients with understandable information of the medical risks and benefits of the different dialysis treatment methods, nephrologists, renal social workers, and associated professionals should be willing and able to discuss the temporal demands that each treatment may entail. The choice between institutional time and personal time can thereby be made part of the decision.

Surgery. Surgery is one of the most anxious events in a person's hospitalization. Here the disparity between the patient's and the institution's time is greatly amplified by the patient's need for calm and deliberate assurance from the staff, and the institution's requirement (or surgeon's requirement) for expeditious time management. The loss of time from anesthesia, and the frequently encountered fear of not waking up at all, also give surgery a special temporal quality for some patients.

To make surgery more humane and to bridge some of the time incongruities, a number of hospitals utilize preoperative and postoperative visits by the Operating Room (O.R.) staff. A day or two prior to the operation, an O.R. nurse will answer questions the patient may have. The O.R. nurse will also say that he/she will be available at any time for any further information the patient might want before the operation—often the same ground is gone over repeatedly, without regard for the time that it takes to reassure the patient.

Although this may seem to be only a small gesture, many patients and staff report that the approach helps to reduce anxiety and convey an impression that the hospital is flexible and humane, rather than a place for assembly line medicine. In addition, such procedures also reduce the patients' perceptions of the duration of waiting time before surgery. In many fields it is commonly held that intervals of waiting time are judged to be shorter if this time is meaningfully occupied.

However meritorious, visits by O.R. staff that are designed to transmit information about what will (or may) happen before, during, and after surgery merely include the patient as a passive participant. Hospitals rarely inquire as to patient or family preferences for surgery times, but concentrate instead on maximizing the flow of patients through limited surgical suites and recovery rooms in the least amount of time. Although no systematic research has ever been done to ascertain the value of including noninstitutional concerns in time-of-day surgical scheduling, priorities will probably differ for young, old, or extremely anxious patients.

To illustrate the limited perspective commonly adopted in surgical scheduling, consider how one group of health care researchers investigated priority rules for determining the daily surgery schedule in a hospital with five surgical suites and twelve recovery rooms.[12] The purpose of the investigation was to determine (via computer simulation methodology) which of five different priority rules would result in the lowest average time of completion of daily surgical loads. The priority rules were:

- Random order—the hospital's current practice.
- Those requiring recovery rooms scheduled first.
- Those requiring estimated longest surgeries and recovery rooms first; otherwise longest surgeries first.
- Estimated longest surgeries first.
- A specific operation first; others next; those not requiring recovery rooms last.

Results from the study showed improvements in performance with any of the nonrandom rules. The best priority rule was one that scheduled surgeries in order of estimated length of time (longest first). As a consequence, it was projected that time saved could result in personnel reductions of one registered nurse and one O.R. technician.

It is indicative that none of the priority rules incorporated any element of patient preferences. Would every patient prefer to be scheduled for surgery at 7 A.M.? Would some prefer to be scheduled later in the day so that they could sleep overnight in the recovery room? What is the effect on an extremely anxious child or adult of delaying a simple surgery until late in the day? How much less efficient would the schedule be if it attempted to meet patient preferences when they were expressed? These questions may not even be important, but until they are raised we cannot know.

Most importantly, scheduling schemes such as those mentioned, with or without incorporating expressed patient preferences, are probably doomed to failure because of the interests of surgeons and associated hospital medical staffs. Indeed, one might reasonably assume that current surgical scheduling practice, which in the research discussed above yielded a random ordering, always reflects a mixture of the preferences of surgeons, anesthesiologists, operating room nurses, technicians, and administrative staff who are assigned scheduling responsibilities, and is not randomly determined.

Well-managed hierarchical organizations rarely (if ever) use random decision rules for planning activities. Priorities are established or derived as a consequence of the interests of the most powerful groups in the hierarchy. Administrative priority rules, or even a true random ordering, may serve as a means of conflict resolution within professional groups when competing interests are involved. But most often, lower echelon ancillary personnel, equipment, and other resources, as well as patients, are usually shifted or diverted to accommodate the special temporal interests of the professional groups in control. When it comes to surgeries, surgeons as a rule do not hesitate to exert their leverage to obtain the operating schedules they desire. Administrators value the revenue surgeons generate for their hospitals and act accordingly in honoring scheduling requests. O.R. staff follow suit, with many "burning out" or becoming disaffected due to the rigors of intensely tight schedules. Patients are least able to express their preferences because they are never asked.

In surgical scheduling, an appropriate ethical position would minimally include giving weight to patient preferences that are based upon nontrivial considerations. Knowing what is nontrivial requires systematic investigation and research rather than untested assumptions. Knowing what weight to place upon patient preferences as opposed to surgeon, medical staff, or administrative preferences should be a matter of collaborative judgment. In the short run, perhaps all that is possible is some explication to patients as to why priorities are established as they are. Real or perceived inequities are often best dealt with by acknowledging their existence and confronting them directly.

Prevention.   To the individual, time is a scarce resource. Within the limits of knowledge of expected future events, individuals face the problem of allocating time in an efficient manner. A major decision is the allocation of time between work and leisure. Work time is linked to socially recognized and institutionally compensated productive activity, and leisure time to unproductive activity. Unproductive activity encompasses all time devoted to consumption and also includes time physically and mentally necessary to insure that work functions can be carried out in the future. Time devoted to renewing and protecting one's health and longevity as a producer is therefore a matter of individual choice, but is strongly constrained by social arrangements requiring work. These constraints lead to a class-dependent orientation to time and to health preservation, and requires further discussion.

Powerlessness associated with lower-class work activities, and life in general, produces a class-differentiated attitude to time allocation. Lower-class individuals who are frequently faced with an indefinite, vague, or diffuse future are not sufficiently motivated by the long-term rewards or punishments related to personal health maintenance. An environment of unemployment, hunger, and physical violence precipitates a time orientation that is characterized by a quick succession of tension and release. By contrast, upper-class individuals view the world in terms of long time sequences and usually can be expected to allocate more time and effort to personal preventive health care actions, such as regular exercise, balanced diets, and limited alcohol consumption.

It is revealing that traditional economists' theories implicitly support a disproportionate class-oriented time allocation to health prevention, since they propose that the social value of an individual's time is related to the person's wage rate.[13] By this accounting, a week spent in a hospital by the president of one of America's leading companies might be as much as one thousand times as socially costly as that of one of the president's production workers. Although it is implausible that an executive would, or could, proportionately spend that much more time in preventing illness than the production worker, we can, thereby, infer a powerful force in favor of maintaining the health of the industrial leader.

Industry has, in fact, taken the lead in implementing health assessment screening education and physical fitness programs for its managers and important personnel. Most large corporations have exercise programs for their executives—some of them in elaborately equipped company facilities that are in use throughout the regular business day. Only the Chinese and Japanese seem to believe that ordinary production workers deserve breaks in the work day for organized physical fitness. Needless to say, no one has organized the poor or unemployed into such programs, although they might benefit the most.

The value conflict that is implied in a discussion of activities designed to provide health maintenance is not one that pits individual patient against provider, but one that is based upon disenfranchisement of those who are unable to value future time because of present time pressures and ignorance. The relative allocation of societal resources favoring curative care over prevention further amplifies this conflict. When coupled with the existence of forms of universal catastrophic health insurance, lower-class improvidence or ignorance can thereby benefit a medical establishment geared to curative care. Unfortunately, the dismantling of proven federal health care prevention initiatives, such as the Special Supplemental Food Program for Women, Infants, and Children (WIC) and Food Stamp Programs, will only exacerbate these class-differentiated trends. Current political rhetorical emphasis on moderating self-imposed risks falls on deaf ears in the ghetto. The appropriate ethical position is to increasingly direct our time and energies to improving methods of preventive medicine, unless we are prepared to face heavy social and financial consequences. Specifically, we need to engage in research activities designed to address the following questions:

- What factors contribute to socioeconomic class-differentiated behavior, attitudes, and values toward time spent in health prevention activities?

- Which of these factors are subject to change without infringing upon the freedom of individuals to live as they please or without encouraging the further medicalization of society?

- What types of educational, marketing, or institutional programs and incentives are most effective in increasing the amount of time devoted to health maintenance among disadvantaged stratas of society?

As long as society values the provision of curative care for all of its members, and mutalizes the cost of this care through health insurance, it will be driven by economic necessity alone to value health prevention for all of its members. Corporations that "invest" in health prevention programs for their employees may be motivated by good intentions, but they are chiefly interested in protecting or increasing their productive human capital and avoiding unnecessary escalations in health insurance costs. Similarly, as improvidence and ignorance influence personal life-styles and thereby affect the overall social balance sheet through rising health care expenditures, an increased emphasis on health prevention becomes necessary. The manner in which one strata of society allocates time for health prevention thus becomes a concern for all.

FUTURE WORK

Health care activities, like all events, occupy physical time. They are unique, however, in that the practice of medicine gives those who deliver it tremendous powers over people by offering means to modify and extend human time. Most of life's events and temporal priorities are not subject to medical intervention, but when medicine does get involved we therefore expect it to do so expeditiously, equitably, and with great sensitivity to individual needs and expectations. Priorities and schedules that are set arbitrarily, for professional "convenience" or according to accidents of birth, class, or geography of the patient, tend to value human time, and hence life itself, differentially. Moreover, health services that are provided without giving weight to significant and appropriate personal time preferences deny patient autonomy.

Individuals will have to submit to institutional time on many occasions, but there should be ample justification for this requirement. Well-managed and humane health institutions will doubtless be able to incorporate more patient preferences through imaginative use of their resources. The demise of block scheduling in ambulatory care, the growth of preadmission testing, variable meal and discharge times, around-the-clock hospital visiting hours, and ambulatory surgery—all within relatively recent years—suggest that greater institutional flexibility is possible and can serve the interests of patients and health providers alike. Further advances in medical instrumentation, pharmaceuticals, surgical procedure, and health maintenance activities will reduce hospital admissions rates and lengths of stay and therefore institutional intervention. The sophisticated hospital information system of the future will be able to coordinate hospital resources while explicitly incorporating individual patient preferences.

For the present, those interested in the ethics of medical care might divert a portion of their attention away from the flashy subjects that command headlines or notoriety, and begin to look instead at the everyday practice of medicine and how priorities and schedules are established and patients' preferences are determined and attended to. Kidney dialysis, surgical scheduling, and health prevention activities are but three isolated areas where value conflicts relating to temporal priorities are easily revealed. Attention might also be given to the priorities of other classes of patients (e.g., geriatric, terminally ill, intensive care, pediatric, and severely disabled), to patients of different ethnic or cultural backgrounds, to patients awaiting transplants or major surgical intervention, or simply to individuals seeking primary care. The objective of these endeavors should be directed toward extending the "perception" and concern of the health provider and the health institution beyond the tissue and functioning organ, to the entire person.[14]

NOTES TO CHAPTER 4

1. Jean L. Marx, "Sudden Death: Strategies for Prevention," *Science* 195 (1977): 39–41.

2. A.T. Beck and A.J. Rush, "Cognitive Approaches to Depression and Suicide," in G. Servan, ed., *Cognitive Defects in the Development of Mental Illness* (New York: Brunner/Mazel, 1978), pp. 235–57.

3. Margaret A. Newman, "Movement Tempo and the Experience of Time," *Nursing Research* 25 (1976): 273–279.

4. Rhode A. Hendricks, *Classical Gods and Heroes* (New York: Frederick Ungar, 1972).

5. Michel Foucoult, *The Birth of the Clinic* (New York: Pantheon Books, 1973).

6. *Ibid.*, p. xviii.

7. Henry E. Sigerist, *Medicine and Human Welfare* (New Haven: Yale University Press, 1941).

8. Leonard W. Doob, *Patterning of Time* (New York: Yale University Press, 1971).

9. Gina Bari Kolata, "NMC Thrives Selling Dialysis," *Science* 208 (1980): 379–382.

10. Thomas Manis and Eli A. Friedman, "Dialytic Therapy for Irreversible Uremia," *The New England Journal of Medicine* 301 (1979): 1260–1265.
11. Edmund D. Lowrie and C.L. Hampers, "The Success of Medicare's End-Stage Renal-Dialysis Program," *The New England Journal of Medicine* 305 (1981): 434–438.
12. N.K. Kwak, P.J. Kuzdrall, and Homer H. Schmitz, "The GPSS Simulation of Scheduling Policies for Surgical Patients," *Management Science* 22 (1976): 982–989.
13. G.S. Becker, "A Theory of the Allocation of Time," *Economic Journal* 75 (1965): 493–517.
14. I am indebted to Bart Gruzalski and Sharon B. Young for their suggestions.

5 THE LAST EPIDEMIC
Medical Responsibility and Thermonuclear War

Andrew Jameton and Christine K. Cassel

At conferences attended by hundreds of physicians, H. Jack Geiger, M.D., Professor of Community Medicine at City College of New York, describes the impossibility of a meaningful medical response to thermonuclear war. In a calculation based on optimistic predictions of the numbers of critically wounded survivors of nuclear attack on any major city, and on the probable number of physicians surviving such an attack, he estimates approximately 1700 acutely injured persons to each functioning doctor, It would take 8 to 14 days to see each patient for 10 minutes if the doctors worked 20 hours a day. Ten minutes would, of course, be inadequate time to care for the injured, whose afflictions would include massive burns, shock, hemorrhage, and acute radiation sickness. Furthermore, virtually all hospital facilities and supplies necessary to intervene effectively in such injuries would have been destroyed.[1]

The physicians who sit in these audiences are receiving continuing medical education credits for attending these conferences, which are sponsored by Physicians for Social Responsibility (PSR), whose objective it is to inform the public about the dangers of nuclear war. The organization was formed in the early 1960s and was revived in 1979 under the leadership of Helen Caldicott. PSR has been conducting a national series of symposia on the medical consequences of nuclear weapons, and is supporting international physicians' associations aimed at reducing the danger of nuclear war. Several articles on the subject have appeared in medical journals.[2]

PSR claims that physicians have a unique and special responsibility to help prevent nuclear war. This is clearly a statement about the professional responsibilities of physicians, and as such is subject to philosophical and ethical discourse. Although it may seem obvious that everyone, including physicians, would be opposed to nuclear war, it is unusual to include in a statement of medical responsibility a matter so far removed from daily clinical activities. Nevertheless, we believe that PSR presents a strong and forceful argument for medical responsibility with regard to nuclear war and that this argument withstands common objections. So far, there has been no systematic statement by PSR of its position, nor has there been an analysis of the extent of physician responsibility in this area. As membership in PSR grows and as increasing public attention is focused in this area, we feel that such an analysis is both timely and important to the delineation of the appropriate role of the medical profession.

Do physicians have a special responsibility to prevent nuclear war? Hiatt has responded affirmatively:

> . . . any nuclear war would inevitably cause death, disease, and suffering of epidemic proportions and without effective intervention. That reality, in turn, leads to the same conclusion we have reached for such contemporary epidemics as lung cancer and heart disease: prevention is essential for effective control.
>
> . . . [W]here treatment of a given disease is ineffective, or where costs are insupportable, attention must be given to prevention. Both conditions apply to the effects of nuclear war—treatment programs would be virtually useless, and the costs would be staggering.[3]

Hiatt's statement highlights part of an argument that can be outlined as follows:

1. Physicians have a special and central moral responsibility to treat disease and to reduce mortality.
2. A large-scale nuclear war would cause death and illness on a massive and unprecedented scale.
3. A large-scale nuclear war is probable in the decades ahead.
4. Prevention is the only way to reduce mortality from an incurable fatal disease.

5. Physicians would be wholly unable to treat effectively a significant portion of death and illness expected in a large-scale nuclear war.

6. Therefore, physicians have a central and urgent moral responsibility to help prevent nuclear war.

The force of this argument can be appreciated better when each of the premises is discussed in detail.

1. *Physicians have a Special and Central Moral Responsibility to Treat Disease and to Reduce Mortality.* This premise stands for a list of responsibilities commonly accepted by physicians. *First*, it is generally held that physicians have responsibilities arising from their special knowledge of medicine and medical practice. When medical knowledge is important for public health, physicians have traditionally held that promulgating medical knowledge is one of their important responsibilities. Thus, where physicians have knowledge not available to others of dangers to health, they have a positive duty to alert those concerned.

Second, physicians have a host of social responsibilities arising from their commitment to patient care. Their first responsibility is for the care of those patients with whom they already have a physician-patient relationship. Where it appears important and effective in order to maintain the health of their patients, physicians regularly attempt to influence their habits and environment to help them gain control over chronic and acute illnesses. They do so even though some health problems arise as much from behavioral and social causes as they do from biological causes..

Some may object that the physician-patient relationship is a voluntary and limited one, and that so far, not many patients have gone to their physicians for protection from nuclear war. The following considerations mitigate this charge of paternalism:

1. When a great danger to one's patient comes to light through medical research, a physician has a responsibility to communicate such risks to his or her patients. Physicians who treated pregnant women with diethylstilbesterol had an obligation to notify those women that their daughters were at risk for vaginal adenocarcinoma.

2. PSR physicians have not coerced patients, attempted to limit their freedom, or imposed on them in a way suggesting force.

Their actions have been directed entirely toward public information. At one hospital in the San Francisco Bay area, physicians circulate a mimeographed sheet on the problems of nuclear war to patients. Although traditional medical authority may lend weight to these communications, physicians place no pressure on patients to behave in any particular way.

3. Opposing nuclear war also has some kinship with such problems as child abuse and occupational health hazards. In such cases, one's patient is endangered primarily by the actions of others and is, to some degree, helpless to resist. Although patients may not contract with physicians to protect them individually from workplace toxins, and children may not ask to be protected from child abuse, physicians still have a responsibility to assist patients in resisting the force of these problems.

It can be objected that since activities involved in resisting nuclear weapons are primarily political, nuclear war is therefore not a medical concern. However, issues cannot be ruled out a medical concerns because they have political aspects. Cancer, smoking, prenatal and child care, communicable disease, and occupational safety all have political aspects. Yet physicians have made a clear commitment to be involved in these matters and the major health dimensions of them rightly remain an important concern of health professionals.

Third, a concern for the health of the public at large has gradually become established as an important responsibility of the medical profession. The specialty of public health medicine has resulted partly from the recognition that physicians can appropriately provide certain kinds of health care for large masses of persons. This is one of the most political areas of medical practice, because it is often necessary to affect social processes in order to establish preventive or screening programs. Public health activities are often supported by local, state, and federal governments. Thus, many of the public health functions of medicine can be accomplished by specialized institutions and professionals. However, where there is no established practice to address a problem, it falls upon the medical profession at large to bring urgent health problems to light.

2. *A Large-scale Nuclear War Would Cause Death and Illness on a Massive and Unprecedented Scale.* It is impossible to assess accurately how many lives might be lost in a large-scale nuclear war; it all

depends on how large the nuclear war is. Many have observed that the megatonnage now stockpiled could exterminate all life on the surface of the earth several times over. More conservative estimates rest on a scenario constituted by an exchange by the United States and the U.S.S.R. of their warheads ready for immediate firing. The National Security Council, for example, published a rough estimate of 140 million immediate casualties in the United States.[4] This compares with 1 million American casualties in all past wars in which the United States has participated. Acute casualties would be followed by long-term casualties, which are inestimable. These would arise from such sources as fallout, residual radiation, infection, poisoning of food and water supplies, effects on atmospheric conditions, social disruption, and psychiatric calamities. Some scientists doubt that anyone would survive. If some did, it would be in a bleak, poisonous, and desperate world. There would be little hope of establishing a level of civilization similar to what we have now.

Focus on survival is, of course, understandable in the face of such imposing figures. We want to hope that somehow we will pull through in any circumstance. However, this focus overlooks the public health problem posed by a large-scale nuclear war. Whatever the number of survivors, injury and death of hundreds of millions of people is a major medical problem. These casualties cannot be set aside in our minds as a special kind of casualty not to be counted in medical consideration: they are the very same people who are currently under treatment for hypertension, diabetes, and so on. Nuclear war is a health risk to each physician's patients, and would create enormous numbers of new patients for the few remaining physicians.

3. *A Large-scale Nuclear War is Probable in the Decades Ahead.* The estimate of the probability is, of course, extremely uncertain. There are good reasons for gloomy prognostications. In the 1950s, the public experienced great concern over the potential dangers of an all-out thermonuclear war. Since that time, the total megatonnage of atomic weaponry and the variety of delivery systems has increased greatly. Recent estimates find approximately 40,000 nuclear devices, and that number is increasing rapidly.[5] Moreover, the number of countries possessing weapons has increased. At the same time, hazardous world conflicts continue, and our historical experience of war suggests that it is only a matter of time until these weapons are used. George Kistiakowsky, former head of the Manhattan Project's ex-

plosive division, and scientific advisor to Presidents Eisenhower, Kennedy, and Johnson, stated, "I personally think that the likelihood for an initial use of nuclear warheads is really quite great between now and the end of this century, which is only 20 years hence."[6] The extensive and highly responsive systems prepared for "mutual assured destruction," and held in hair-trigger balance by the United States and the U.S.S.R., combined with more recent developments for counterforce strategies and plans for tactical use of nuclear weapons, would make restrained use of these weapons improbable.

Since nuclear war is not a certainty, our worry over it should be diminished in proportion to its likelihood. Thus, we attempted a crude estimate of what measure of concern it deserves. We asked: How many lives would prevention of nuclear war be likely to save as compared, for example, to finding a cure for cancer? Using Kistiakowsky's 20-year perspective, we estimated roughly how many deaths to expect from cancer in the next 20 years and compared it to the Security Council estimate. About 7.5 million U.S. cancer deaths can be expected in the next 20 years as compared to the rough estimate of 140 million from nuclear war. We calculate that a probability of about one chance in 20 of nuclear war 20 years from now would yield an expected death figure (expected deaths equals number of deaths times probability of deaths) like that from 20 years of cancer. Pushing the cost-benefit approach further, we calculated figures for expected life-years lost from cancer and nuclear war (expected life-years lost equals average life expectancy at age of death times deaths times probability of deaths). Twenty years of cancer would yield about 110 million life-years lost as compared to about 6.03 billion life-years lost in a nuclear war. Thus, the probability of nuclear war at the end of 20 years would have to be about one chance in 50 to reduce the level of concern to that of cancer. If nuclear war is probable in the next 20 years, this calculation suggests that it warrants a much greater level of concern than cancer.[7]

4. *Prevention is the Only Way to Reduce Mortality From an Incurable Fatal Disease.* It is only a practical generalization that it is better to prevent trouble than to wait for it to come. Before we can set a priority on prevention, we need to ask some questions about what is to be prevented and what are the benefits of a course of prevention.

We have already begun to establish that nuclear war would cause harm on an incredible scale; that it would not only cause incurable disease, but incurable disease on such a scale as to be possibly geno-cidal. We also need to consider, however, what other claims are being made on our attention. We must consider the moral claims of those who are already ill and compare them with those who may become ill in the future. Since medicine is a compassionate enterprise, the claims on physicians of those who now have cancer are stronger than those who may have cancer in the future. PSR does not suggest that physicians should desert patient care in favor of campaigns against nuclear war. The danger of nuclear war is, however, great enough that physicians should add a concern for it to their schedules.

The costs of prevention are also irrelevant. They are, of course, uncertain, and very much affected by the means chosen. Since great changes would be required to avert the hazard of nuclear war, phy-sicians cannot speak to the costs of prevention. They can speak to the personal costs of their own involvement in efforts to prevent it. The worst outcome is that physicians would spend great energy in order to avert the hazard, and yet nuclear war would take place any-way. The best outcome—that the risk of nuclear war be greatly re-duced—seems so attractive that many physicians would feel satisfied in that result even if it cost them a great deal of personal sacrifice and suffering.

The critical consideration is whether prevention is possible. Is there any reason to think that activity by physicians can help to prevent nuclear war? The present and continuing threat of nuclear weapons was the result of concerted efforts of groups of human beings and their institutions. We have no good reason to think that countervail-ing efforts by other groups of human beings *cannot* be effective in preventing nuclear war. Moreover, organized opposition to nuclear war may be *necessary* to prevent it. Physicians may even have some special power in coping with this problem. Instead of appearing as a threat to autonomy, the traditional authority of the physician adds weight to the PSR message on nuclear war. Evgueni Chazof, Leonid Brezhnev's personal physician and a cardiologist, for example, ex-plained why he thought international physicians for the prevention of nuclear war might have more impact than other groups: "They do not have access to people's hearts, like we physicians do."[8] More-over, physicians are familiar with the phenomenon of denial in the face of a terminal diagnosis. The denial of the true risk of the horrors of nuclear destruction may have a useful function in making it pos-sible for all of us to go about our daily lives, and in that sense it is an adaptive psychological mechanism. Such denial operating at the level of those who make strategic military and political policy is, however, extremely maladaptive.[9] Bringing the horrible facts about the medical consequences of nuclear weapons and nuclear war to light in public discussions may seem to be a cruel awakening, but it is in fact the first step toward the only realistic mechanism for coping with the problem—prevention.

Physicians are also sensitive to the role ambivalence plays in supporting chronic health problems. In spite of great numbers of people killed by nuclear war, some hope that we could create out of that ruin a better life for survivors than is possible in our present world. Many people hate certain things about the world as it exists now: the earth is being paved over; rooms are growing smaller; the air and vegetables are less palatable; resources are short; and contaminants are more common. We cannot see clearly how to bring industrialization under the control of humane principles. Sudden destruction of our civilization would solve many of these problems. Certain "survivalists" have said they are eager for a nuclear holocaust, certain that they will survive and that less desirable elements of society will not.[10]

Just as the actual expectations of nuclear war are an important motivation for medical concern about it, presentation of these facts by physicians is essential to counteract denial and ambivalence. As pointed out by Hiatt, Lown, and others, the survivalist vision is merely a fantasy. If more than 140 million people die instantly in the United States, you and I will likely be among those millions. If we do not die, we will almost certainly be among the critically injured. If we remain alive, our lives would be a desperate struggle. The epidemics of disease, cancer, starvation, and trauma could not easily be considered better than immediate death. Our present technological achievements support us so well that we would be unsuited for and unskilled at rediscovering forgotten techniques for more primitive lives. Moreover, we would not be relieved of scarcity and pollution. Our world would be smeared with ashen death, scorched, poisoned, and laced with radioactivity. To imagine escape from these consequences, we have to turn to science fiction: orbital burn units or the escape of the few to colonize another planet. These fantasies do not address the basic health problems of the casualties.

5. Physicians Would Be Wholly Unable to Treat Effectively a Significant Portion of Death and Illness Expected in a Large-scale Nuclear War.   The impotence of the medical profession to respond to nuclear casualties has proved the most effective and moving consideration to medical audiences. Since medical institutions are concentrated in large cities—prime target areas—nuclear war would result in a disproportionately large destruction of health personnel and equipment. The sheer numbers of casualties would make useful treatment virtually impossible. This perception is heightened by present technological development in medicine. An all-out attempt to save the life of a single burn patient requires massive resources.[11] That level of response to millions of persons is out of the question, even with undamaged medical capacity. Little could be done by physicians and other health workers in Hiroshima and Nagasaki to comfort the dying, and for these cities there was outside help available. In the case of large-scale nuclear war, there would be no outside help.

Nuclear war, unlike conventional war, would prevent physicians from fulfilling their responsibilities. It is one thing to hear that we will die; it is another to be told that we will not be able to live meaningfully or to do what we are morally obligated to do.[12] Since physicians are a key element in society's humane response to suffering, the inability of physicians to perform their duty is of great social significance. Civil defense efforts only serve to create the illusion that significant survival is possible, and so it is important for physicians to inform the public that feasible sheltering, evacuation, and medical plans would be unlikely to enhance survival in any meaningful sense of the word.

6. Therefore, Physicians Have a Central and Urgent Moral Responsibility To Help Prevent Nuclear War.   We believe that the premises of this argument are sound, and that the considerations in favor of an important physician responsibility to work for the prevention of nuclear war far outweigh the objections. We also believe that the premises strongly support the conclusion, even though some people are uncomfortable with it. Some feel that physicians, if opposed to nuclear war, should do so out of opposition to all forms of warfare. They are afraid that those who oppose nuclear war might fail to oppose a conventional or technologically inventive war of great destructiveness. Since we can wage war without nuclear weapons, PSR's position seems to suggest that a medically sound form of war is possible. But this is a separate question. First, to argue that physicians also have a responsibility to oppose war in general does not negate their responsibility to oppose nuclear war. More importantly, however, conventional war has permitted some expression of the humane response to suffering as a result of it. Many who are opposed to nuclear war accept that aggression is an intrinsic aspect of most human societies. The force of the PSR argument arises because nuclear weapons present a quantitative difference of such magnitude that it becomes a qualitative difference. Since physicians are concerned about a quantity of destruction greater than that which has been conveived before, resisting the further manufacture and deployment of nuclear weapons need not express an especially idealistic position. The narrow focus on nuclear weapons strengthens PSR's argument: Even minimal humanitarianism requires active opposition to development of nuclear weapons.

Some object that concern for nuclear war is not a unique responsibility of physicians, but that is a concern for everyone. Nuclear war would mean an end to modern music, publishing, biological research, movies, football, roadside fruitstands, public transit, and so on. Don't people working in these areas also have responsibilities to fulfill which nuclear war would prevent?

It would not nullify our argument if it turned out that the responsibility to help prevent nuclear war is a widespread one. Certainly other health care workers who have clinical and social responsibilities similar to physicians, such as nurses, have similar responsibilities with regard to nuclear war. Together with these other health care professionals, physicians have special responsibilities beyond those working in other areas. Health professionals have special knowledge of the risks of nuclear war and also play an important role in dealing with its consequences. Moreover, the inability of most of us to fulfill our duties after nuclear war would arise primarily from health problems about which the health professions have a special responsibility. The first premise of the argument speaks to the concern of health professionals much more than it does to musicians and transit workers. Other arguments based on the loss of music and transit could be addressed to the people working in those areas. Although such arguments are important, the central relevance of life and health to all of us gives special urgency to the argument focused on the responsibilities of health professionals.

The argument is focused largely on the health professions as a whole, and not on particular professionals. PSR is not suggesting that all physicians and nurses should cancel rounds and take to the streets. Nuclear war is primarily a concern of the health professions as a collective whole. To express this collective responsibility, it is only required that a substantial number of health professionals be involved, that is, enough to be efficacious, and that professional associations and institutions incorporate a concern with these issues.

THE RESPONSIBILITIES OF BIOETHICISTS WITH REGARD TO NUCLEAR WAR

Bioethicists spend so much time working in areas of subtle or complex distinctions that it sometimes seems that there are few simple moral arguments. The argument above is offered as an example of a straightforward and sound moral argument. We feel that the argument is strong and convincing, even though it draws a conclusion indirectly related to standard aspects of medical practice. We also believe that the argument shows the importance of conventional practice in appreciating arguments in ethics. The responsibility to be concerned with nuclear war does not arise out of purely philosophical considerations. The argument occurs against the background commitments of medical practice. It says, in effect, that if physicians accept ordinary notions of social responsibility in medical practice, then they also should accept responsibility to be concerned with the threat of nuclear war.

We are also concerned with the ethical responsibilities of bioethicists. We believe that it is important for bioethicists to go beyond identification of dilemmas and exploration of uncertain areas of ethics in the health sciences. Bioethicists also have a responsibility to bring to the attention of ethicists and health professionals clear and important moral arguments as they come to light. The professional ethicist is an explorer, not a propagandist. But in the work of exploration, ethicists come across moral wrongs that need righting, or compelling and important moral points of view. It is impossible in good conscience for an ethicist to maintain a purely exploratory point of view. We believe the argument above is valid and important enough that bioethicists as teachers and consultants in the health professions have a responsibility to join in efforts to prevent a nuclear war.

NOTES TO CHAPTER 5

1. H. Jack Geiger, "Addressing Apocalypse Now and the Effects of Nuclear Warfare as a Public Health Concern," *American Journal of Public Health* 70 (1980): 958–961.

2. See, for example, *Ibid.*, F. Barnaby, "World Arsenals in 1980," *Bulletin of the Atomic Scientists* 36 (1980): 9–14; and Jerome D. Frank, "The Nuclear Arms Race – Sociopsychological Aspects," *American Journal of Public Health* 70 (1980): 950–952.

3. Howard H. Hiatt, "Preventing the Last Epidemic," *Journal of the American Medical Association* 244 (1980): 2314–2315.

4. *Presidential Review Memorandum* no. 10, U.S. National Security Council (June, 1977).

5. Barnaby, "World Arsenals in 1980," pp. 9–14.

6. Quoted by Jonathan A. Leonard, "Danger: Nuclear War," *Harvard Magazine* (November–December 1980): 21–25.

7. We used United States 1976 figures for overall population cancer deaths grouped by age, life expectancy, and so forth, but ignored such things as population growth. Our statistics are based on figures from the Department of Health, Education, and Welfare, *Facts of Life and Death* (PHS79–1222) (Washington, D.C.: Government Printing Office, 1978).

8. *San Francisco Chronicle*, 26 March 1981.

9. Frank, "The Nuclear Arms Race," pp. 950–952.

10. P.F. Kluge, "Hunkering Down: Survivalism," *GEO* 3 (September 1981): 123–140.

11. John D. Constable, "Surgical Problems Among Survivors," *The Bulletin of the Atomic Scientists* 37 (1981): 22–25.

12. Albert Camus, *The Plague* (New York: Modern Library, Inc., 1976).

II CONFRONTING ETHICAL ISSUES

Ethical issues in the delivery of personal health care services are debated and resolved through the activities of lawyers, patient advocates, providers, administrators, and patients themselves. The four chapters in this section deal with the questions of who should be involved in resolving medical-ethical dilemmas and whose decisions are to carry the most weight. These chapters show that the arena in which resolutions are attempted, and the parties involved, strongly influence the scope of the debate and its eventual outcome.

In "The Emerging Stowaway: Patient Rights in the 1980s" George Annas advocates continued establishment of strong minimum standards to protect patients against potential abuses of medical providers. Such standards, with the force of law behind them, already dramatically affect the every-day practice of medicine for all hospitalized patients. Annas's expanded five-point "Rights Agenda" would further limit physician and hospital discretion, while giving the patient strengthened recourse in the courts. His analysis of recent attacks on the patients' rights movement also indicates that many physicians continue to oppose, directly and indirectly, any diminution of their power.

John Paris next examines the special case of protecting the rights and personal preferences of terminally ill patients and demonstrates how intervention by the courts can lead to torturous arguments, costly proceedings, and suffering for patients and their advocates. In his "Medical Ethics, The Courts, and Death with Dignity," Paris holds that the court system is not the best place to center ultimate decisions on life and death matters. He places less faith in lawyers and legal proceedings than George Annas and argues for respecting the wishes of patients, their families, and their advocates.

In the next chapter, "The Geriatric Patient: Ethical Issues in Care and Treatment," Ruth Macklin helps to clarify what we know and do not know about dealing with geriatric and terminally ill patients, establishing their mental competency, and protecting their rights. She points to the growing number of chronically ill patients over 65 that physicians, hospitals, and nursing homes must treat, and how we are often unprepared to understand and meet their physical or psychological needs. Her primary goal is to enhance the quality of life of this special class of patients; for example, by using the "social model" in place of the "medical model" in setting policies for nursing homes and geriatric facilities. If her general objective can be attained, the likelihood of legal interventions would be reduced, and ethical questions would arise less frequently.

The final chapter in this section examines the crucial role that nurses can have in protecting the rights and quality of life of all classes of patients. As executors of physician orders, overseers of physician performance, and round-the-clock participants in the practice of medicine, nurses become involved in a multitude of ethical conflicts. Andrew Jameton begins his "Nurses and Moral Distress in the Hospital" with an examination of the responsibilities and options of nurses as they confront a series of cases that demonstrate a surgeon's incompetency, an incompetency that is not immediately evident in any of the cases taken singly. In his practical essay, Jameton offers specific guidelines for nurses when they believe that their rights or those of their patients are being abrogated.

The chapters in this section may lead one to ask whether ethical dilemmas arising in the delivery of personal medical services might be foreseen or forestalled before they consume valuable human resources, impose unnecessary suffering, or progress to even more severe confrontations. Anticipation and early resolution of ethical problems is difficult, since the delivery of health services often entails application of imperfect medicine to limitless desires and diverse human values. Moreover, as one dilemma gets resolved, another frequently gains prominence. But one suggestion that may lead to the early discovery and resolution of ethical issues involves expanding the problem-oriented medical record and treatment plan to incorporate nonclinical issues. To make this operational, persons involved in the delivery of medical services, along with trained bioethicists, patient advocates, and the patients themselves, would routinely evaluate the appropriateness of care in light of the patient's needs and desires. When problems involving ethical conflicts are discovered or are thought likely to occur, a brief entry would be made on the patient's problem-oriented medical record. Actions contemplated or actually taken to resolve the dilemma would similarly be recorded, along with supporting justifications.

The proposal has a number of desirable features:

- Nonclinical outcomes would be given more formal recognition.

- Health providers would learn to use their considerable diagnostic and analytical intellectual skills to determine problems, discuss objectives, reveal constraints, and present alternatives relevant to the patient's *total* welfare.

- The expanded problem-oriented record could influence the course of treatment, as actions taken in the clinical and nonclinical domain are often strongly interdependent.

- The medical record could serve as a basis for concurrent and retrospective reviews of both the quality of care and the quality of caring.

Inclusion of ethical problems in the medical record fulfills both procedural and substantive objectives. If difficult issues must be decided on a case-by-case basis, then they should be approached systematically. Documentation places both procedures and judgments on record where both may be reviewed. Ethical issues are thereby confronted openly, with a clear recognition of the consequences of decisions.

The expanded use of the problem-oriented medical record would help to meet the objectives outlined by the four authors of this section. Such a device would aid in the protection of those patient rights about which George Annas is concerned. John Paris would favor the gathering of relevant information and viewpoints by parties directly involved in life and death decisions. Ruth Macklin, we think, would welcome the active participation of bioethicists and the ability to focus attention on any special class of patients. For nurses facing the serious issues that Andrew Jameton discusses, the record could be used to enhance and protect the quality of care that patients receive.

6 THE EMERGING STOWAWAY
Patients' Rights in the 1980s

George J. Annas

At one point in Edgar Allan Poe's *Narrative of Arthur Gordon Pym of Nantucket*, Pym, who has stowed away in the hold of a whaling vessel, believes he has been abandoned and that the hold will be his tomb. He expressed sensations of "extreme horror and dismay," and "the most gloomy imaginings, in which the dreadful deaths of thirst, famine, suffocation, and premature interment, crowded in as the prominent disasters to be encountered."

It is probably uncommon for hospitalized patients to feel as gloomy as Pym. Nevertheless, installed in a strange institution, separated from friends and family, forced to wear a degrading costume, confined to bed, and attended to by a variety of strangers who may or may not keep the patient informed of what they are doing, the average patient is intimidated and disoriented. Such an atmosphere encourages dependence and discourages the assertion of individual rights.

As the physician-director of Boston's Beth Israel Hospital has warned: "today's hospital stands increasingly to become a jungle, whose pathways to the uninitiated are poorly marked and fraught with danger . . . "[1] In this jungle the notion that patients have rights that demand respect is often foreign.

The movement for enhanced patients' rights is based on two premises: (1) citizens possess certain rights that are not automatically forfeited by entering into a relationship with a physician or health care facility; and (2) most physicians and health care facilities fail to recognize these rights, fail to provide for their protection or assertion, and limit their exercise without recourse.[2]

The primary argument against patients' rights is that patients have "needs" and defining these needs in terms of rights leads to the creation of an unhealthy adversary relationship.[3] It is not, however, the creation of rights, but the disregard of them, that produces adversaries. When provider and patient work together in an atmosphere of mutual trust and understanding, the articulation of rights can only enhance their relationship.

Many issues cannot be resolved entirely within the provider-patient relationship, however. Providers not only have formal relationships with their patients, but also have relationships with other providers, health care institutions, and numerous governmental agencies. A provider's relationship with these institutions and individuals is often a very complex one, and providers often find themselves confused and therefore submissive in cases where they do not understand their own rights or those of their patients.

RIGHTS IN HEALTH CARE

In most instances, both the health care provider *and* the patient will be better off if the status of the law regarding both patient *and* provider rights is understood, and the means of change or challenge well-delineated.[4] I would go even further. An understanding of the law can be as important to the proper care of patients as an understanding of emergency medical procedures or proper drug dosages. But how are rights to be understood, and how does a person know that he or she has a "right" to something perceived as being desirable to some?

There is formidable literature on rights in the archives of philosophy and jurisprudence. Rather than review it, let me note briefly the thoughts of two relatively recent entrants who have written with great insight. The first is John Rawls. In expounding his *Theory of Justice*,[5] he imagines that a group of men and women come together to form a social contract. These individuals all have ordinary tastes, talents, ambitions, and convictions—but they are all temporarily unaware of their own personality and best interests and must agree to the terms of the contract before awareness of their own identity is restored. The theory postulates that under such circumstances all will agree to two principles: (1) each person shall enjoy the most extensive liberty compatible with a like liberty for all; and (2) inequalities in wealth and power should exist only where they work to the benefit of the worst-off members of society. One could develop an entire system of patients' rights that would rest on these premises. Such a document would be strongly propatient since this group is currently the one that generally lacks rights and is always the group that will be viewed as "worst-off" in the health care setting.

A second approach is suggested by the writings of Ronald Dworkin in his essays *Taking Rights Seriously*.[6] Dworkin notes the great confusion in "rights language" generally created by attributing to it different meanings in different contexts: "In most cases when we say that someone has a right to something, we imply that it would be wrong to interfere with his doing it, or at least that some special grounds are needed for justifying an interference." An example is the right to spend one's money the way one pleases. This is, of course, different from saying that the way one spends one's money, such as gambling it away, is the "right" thing to do, or that there is nothing "wrong" with it. When we speak of patients' rights, this distinction may be critical to understanding what we are talking about. For example, a woman may have a legal right to have an abortion, but she may still consider such a decision "wrong".

Dworkin argues further that there are some rights that can be said to be fundamental in the sense that the government is bound to recognize and protect them. Such rights, which we often denote as "legal rights," and less frequently as "constitutional rights," are generally spelled out in statutes and court decisions. By respecting such rights, the government guarantees to the weakest members of society that they will not be trampled on by the strongest. In Dworkin's words:

> The bulk of the law—that part which defines and implements social, economic, and foreign policy—cannot be neutral. It must state, in its greatest part, the majority's view of the common good. The institution of rights is therefore crucial, because it represents the majority's promise to the minorities that their dignity and equality will be respected. When the divisions among the groups are most violent, then this gesture, if law is to work, must

be most sincere . . . taking individual rights seriously is the one feature that distinguishes law from ordered brutality.[7]

Without going too far afield, one can apply Dworkin's notion directly to health care and note that rights can form a useful means of guaranteeing to defenseless patients that they will be treated with human dignity and respect. Although the health care provider often has the power to deny certain rights almost at will, the provider does this only at the peril of the integrity of the health care system itself.

THE AHA BILL OF RIGHTS

It must strike most people as ironic that the first major health care organization to put forward a patients' bill of rights was the American Hospital Association (AHA), an organization composed primarily of hospital administrators. One would not expect landlords to pen a bill of rights for tenants, police for suspects, or wardens for prisoners. Nor would one reasonably expect that the hospital administrator's view on rights for patients would be the same as either the patient's or society's. Nevertheless, physicians and nurses should be ashamed that the administrators were well out in front of them on this issue. Even though it leaves much to be desired in terms of completeness, specificity, and enforceability, the AHA Bill has tremendous symbolic value in legitimizing the notion of rights in the health care institution.[8] On the other hand, fewer than half of all AHA member hospitals have formally adopted even this bill, and the symbolic victory of the 1970s is currently under attack.

THE ATTACK ON PATIENTS' RIGHTS

Physicians, who perhaps value their own professional autonomy more than any other group, nevertheless devalue it for their own patients. Instead, paternalism is the norm with the majority of physicians believing that the health and continued life of their patients is much more important than their patients' right to self-determination. This belief system not only leads to conflicts with individual patients about their own care, but also to a general view that sees patients' rights as being a luxury item in medicine rather than a necessity.

A few examples illustrate the point. Two particular rights of patients have recently come under attack in the medical literature: access to medical records and informed consent. In an attack on "record reading," four psychiatrists at Boston's Peter Bent Brigham Hospital interviewed the 11 out of 2,500 patients at that hospital in a one year period who asked to see their medical records.[9] It is doubtful that anything of general importance about a patient's reactions to reading their charts can be learned from an uncontrolled, nonblind, clinically impressionistic study of those few individuals who, for whatever reason, buck a system that routinely fails to inform them of their right of access to their records. Nonetheless, the authors' conclusion that such patients have a variety of personality defects, usually manifesting themselves in mistrust of and hostility toward the hospital staff, should not be permitted to go uncontested. In a setting where trusting patients are not routinely told of their right to access, it seems reasonable to assume that only the least trusting or most angry will ask to see their records. To locate the source of mistrust in the patient's personality style or in the stress of illness and hospitalization is to forget, as Dr. Lipsett perceptively suggests, that "the doctor–patient relationship cannot be understood simply in terms of the patient's side of the equation."[10] Altman et al. thus fall into what Professor Robert Burt of the Yale Law School has referred to as "the conceptual trap of attempting to transform two-party relationships, in which mutual self-delineations are inherently confused and intertwined, by conceptually obliterating one party . . ."[11] Thus, it would seem that the ten women who asked to read their charts "to confirm the belief that the staff harbored negative personal attitudes toward them . . ." were correct in the belief; the psychiatrists labelled them "of the hysterical type with demanding, histrionic behavior and emotional over-involvement with the staff."

Altman et al. also seem unaware of the wide variety of settings in which patients have *benefited* from routine record access, and incorrectly assert that there were no strikingly beneficial effects in the two studies they do cite. In the first study, for example, two patients expressed their completely unfounded fear that they had cancer only after their record was reviewed with them, and one pregnant patient noted an incorrect Rh typing that permitted RhoGam to be administered at the time of delivery.[12] In the other study they cite, 50 percent of the patients made some factual correction in the record.[13]

In short, the study seems to have been done and published for the primary purpose of proving that the right to record access is unimportant since it is only exercised by "mentally disturbed" people who are not improved by reading their charts. It fails to prove this, and even if it succeeded, I would still be unwilling to deprive the other 2,489 patients of their right to access in the future. If we believe in individual freedom and the concept of self-determination, we must give all citizens the right to make their *own* decisions and to have access to information that is widely available to those making decisions about them. It is as irrelevant in this connection that 2,489 patients at the Peter Bent Brigham Hospital did not ask to see their records as it is that more 200 million Americans never have had to exercise their right to remain silent when arrested. Rights serve us all, whether we exercise them or not.

The attack on informed consent, which many physicians have long considered a "legal fiction,"[14] most recently surfaced in a study often used to "prove" that informed consent was not an important patients' right in practice, because patients could not remember what they were informed of.[15] The methodology involved interviewing 200 consecutive cancer patients who had consented to chemotherapy, surgery, or radiation therapy for their cancers within 24 hours after they had signed consent forms. Upon questioning, most could not recall the procedure consented to, its major risks, or the alternatives to it. From this the authors conclude that the process is not working and that informed consent itself is suspect. Although this may seem to be a reasonable conclusion (an alternative one is simply that patients have poor recall), it turns out that the authors presumed their major premise. Approximately two-thirds of their sample group (66 percent) opted for radiation therapy. That group signed a consent form that said "the procedure, its risks and benefits and alternatives have been explained to me." Maybe they were, but maybe they were not. The authors did not know, so their entire study was based on a premise that was unsubstantiated. Such a poorly designed study, it seems to me, could only be published if the editors agreed so strongly with the conclusion that they did not even review the methodology.

A perhaps more interesting part of the study asked the patients some general questions about informed consent. The first was, "What are consent forms for?" Approximately 80 percent responded: "To protect the physicians' rights." The authors were upset at this response, but the patients of course were correct. That *is* the primary function of *forms*. If one wants these forms also to protect the patient, three simple steps are necessary: (1) the forms must be complete; (2) they must be in lay language; and (3) the patients must be given a copy of the form and time to think over the information it contains.[16] The reason none of these is usually done is clear: Informed consent is not taken seriously in the hospital setting. It is, like record access, a luxury that is secondary to caring for the medical "needs" of the patient, and besides, it really doesn't matter anyway because patients can't remember anything they've been told . . .

Other significant findings that indicate the extent to which patients understand and appreciate the consent process are: 80 percent thought the forms were necessary; 76 percent thought they contained just the right amount of information; 84 percent understood all or most of the information; 75 percent thought the explanations given were important; and 90 percent said they would try to remember the information contained on the forms. To me, this suggests that the patients surveyed, understood, and appreciated the informed consent process much better than the researchers did. Their data are certainly not flawless, but one can conclude from the data just the opposite of what the researchers did: For almost all patients, informed consent is seen as very important.

Related to this general attack on rights is an attack on the patient population itself. The notion is that the major problems with the health care delivery system are not problems with providers, but with patients. We eat too much, smoke too much, do not exercise enough, take too many risks, and it serves us right if we get sick. The American health care enterprise must deal with a bad class of patients that (on top of everything) now not only wants access to care, but also wants some say in what kind of care is provided! As Lewis Thomas has put it in a related vein, this is becoming folk doctrine about disease. You become ill because of not living right. If you get cancer it is, somehow or other, your own fault. If you didn't cause it by smoking or drinking, or eating the wrong things, it came from allowing yourself to persist with the wrong kind of personality in the wrong environment."[17]

This attitude would be humorous if it was not so pervasive and did not affect patient care so profoundly. Martha Lear has given us some excellent and telling examples in her deeply moving book, *Heartsounds*, that chronicles the final four years of life of her physician-husband who goes through eight operations and eleven hospitalizations during that period. Together they identify the "it's your fault ploy," which means that no matter what goes wrong in the hospital setting, it is the fault of the patient, not the health care system.

> Why did the operation take so long?
> Because you lost so much blood.
> *Not*: Because the surgeon blew it.
> Why do you keep making these tests?
> Because you have a very stubborn infection.
> *Not*: Because I can't diagnose your case.
> Why did I get sick again?
> Because you were very weak.
> *Not*: Because I did not treat you competently the first time.[18]

Dr. Lear is constantly asking himself if he treated patients that way, and usually admits that he did. He suggests that every physician be required to spend at least a week a year in a hospital bed: "That would change some things in a hurry."[19]

AN AGENDA FOR THE 80s

Since patients *do* have rights and *do* want to exercise them, and since the major attacks on the notion of patients' rights have been based on sloppy studies and false premises, the patients' rights movement is likely to gain momentum. Indeed, the 1970s can be most properly viewed as a decade in which the notion of rights has become legitimized through basic education of health care providers to the existence of patients' rights. I suggest that the 1980s will be a decade in which the primary thrust will be working on ways to directly enhance the status of patients in the hospital as a means of humanizing the hospital environment so that patients can have a greater voice in how they are treated.

I suggest the following five point Patients' Rights Agenda for the 1980s:

1. No Routine Procedures
2. Open Access to Medical Records
3. Twenty-Four-Hour-a-Day Visitor Rights
4. Full Experience Disclosure
5. Effective Patient Advocate

1. *No Routine Procedures.* It is all too common for nurses and others to respond to the question, "Why is this being done?" with, "Don't worry, it's routine." This should not be an acceptable response. No procedure should *ever* be performed on a patient because it is routine; it should only be performed if it is *specifically* indicated for that patient. Thus, routine admission tests, routine use of john-nies, routine use of wheelchairs for in-hospital transportation, and routine use of sleeping pills, to name a few notable examples, would be abolished. Use of these procedures means patients are treated as fungible robots rather than individual human beings. These procedures are often demeaning and unnecessary.

2. *Open Access to Medical Records.* Although currently provided for by federal law and many state statutes and regulations, open access to medical records by patients remain difficult, and patients often assert their right to see their records at the peril of being labeled "distrustful" or "trouble-maker." The information in the hospital chart is about the patient and properly belongs to the patient. The patient must have access to it, both to enhance his or her own decisionmaking ability and to make it clear that the hospital is an "open" institution that is not trying to hide things from the patient. Surely if hospital personnel are making decisions about the patient on the basis of information in the chart, the patient also deserves access to the information.

3. *Twenty-Four-Hour-a-Day Visitor Rights.* One of the most important ways to both humanize the hospital and enhance patient autonomy is to ensure that at least one person of the patient's choice has unlimited access to the patient at any time of the day or night. This person should also be permitted to stay with the patient during any procedure (e.g., childbirth, induction of anesthesia), as long as the person does not interfere with the care of other patients.

4. *Full Experience Disclosure.* The most important gain of the past decade has been the almost universal acknowledgment of the need for the patient's informed consent. Nevertheless, some information that is material to the patient's decision is still withheld: the experience of the person doing the procedure.[20] Patients have a right to know if the person asking permission to draw blood, take blood gases, do a bone marrow aspiration, or do a spinal tap has ever per-

formed the procedure before, and if so, what the person's complication rate is. This applies not only to student nurses, but also to board certified surgeons—we all do things for the first time, and not every patient wants to take such an active role in our education.

5. *An Effective Patient Advocate.* Although a patients' bill of rights is necessary, it is not sufficient. Rights are not self-actualizing. Patients are sick and desire relief from pain and discomfort more than they demonstrate a desire to exercise their rights; they are also anxious, and may hold back complaints for fear of retaliation. It is critical that patients have access to a person whose job it is to work *for the patient* to help the patient exercise the rights outlined in the institution's bill of rights. This person should sit in on all major hospital committees that deal with patient care, have authority to obtain medical records for patients, call consultants, launch complaints directly with all members of the hospital, medical, nursing, and administrative staff, and be able to delay discharges. Although there appear to be some successful "patient representatives" that are hired by the hospitals, it is not fair to give them this title since they must represent the hospital, and it is likely that ultimately effective representation can only be obtained by someone who is hired by a consumer group or governmental agency outside of the hospital in which the representative works.

CONCLUSION

We have made a beginning in the long journey toward humanizing the hospital and promoting patient self-determination in it. But more specific measures are needed before patients will be assured that they can effectively exercise their rights in institutional settings.

Like Poe's Arthur Gordon Pym, the notion that patients have rights has survived the days of darkness, isolation, and starvation. It is now generally accepted (although sporadically attacked) and it is up to patients and providers alike to see to it that these rights become a reality for every citizen.

NOTES TO CHAPTER 6

1. M. Rabkin, quoted in G. J. Annas, "The Hospital: A Patient Rights Waste-land, *Civil Liberties Review* (Fall 1974): 11.
2. See generally, G. J. Annas, *The Rights of Hospital Patients* (New York: Avon, 1975).
3. E.G. Margolis, "Conceptual Aspects of a Patient's Bill of Rights," *Connecticut Medicine Supplement* 43, no. 9 (October 1979): 9-11. Also see Ladd, "Legalism and Medical Ethics," in Davis, Hoffmaster, and Shorten, eds., *Contemporary Issues in Biomedical Ethics* (New Jersey, Humana Press, 1978), pp. 1-35.
4. Examples of patient abuse based on provider misunderstanding of the law after the Saikewicz case in Massachusetts are cited in G. J. Annas, "Reconciling Quinlan and Saikewicz: Decision Making for the Terminally Ill Incompetent," *American Journal of Law and Medicine* 4, no. 4. (1979): 367, 387.
5. J. Rawls, *A Theory of Justice* (Cambridge, Mass.: Harvard University Press, 1971).
6. R. Dworkin, *Taking Rights Seriously* (Cambridge, Mass.: Harvard University Press, 1977), p. 188.
7. *Ibid.*, p. 205.
8. Reprinted in Annas, pp. 25-27.
9. J.H. Altman, P. Reich, M.J. Kelly and M.P. Rogers, "Patients Who See Their Medical Record," *New England Journal of Medicine* 302, no. 3 (1980): 169.
10. D. Lipsett, "The Patient and the Record," *New England Journal of Medicine* 302, no. 3 (1980): 167.
11. R. Burt, *Taking Care of Strangers: The Rule of Law in Doctor-Patient Relations* (New York: The Free Press, 1979), p. 43.
12. D.P. Stevens, R. Staff, and I. MacKay, "What Happens When Hospitalized Patients See Their Own Records," *Annals of Internal Medicine* 86 (1977): 474, 476.
13. A. Golodetz, J. Ruess, and R. Milhous, "The Right to Know: Giving the Patient His Medical Record," *Archives of Physical Medicine and Rehabilitation* 57 (1976): 78, 81. And experience under the new record access regulation enacted by the Board of Registration in Medicine indicates that patients want access to their records for a variety of reasons. In the period from October 13, 1978 (when the regulation went into effect), to January 31, 1980, the Medicine Board received more phone calls from consumers asking about the medical records regulation (approximately ten a month) than about any other single issue dealt with by the Board. There were also 33 formal complaints filed concerning record access during this

period. Of this number, almost half (16) needed help from the Board to get their physician to forward a copy of their record directly to another physician. Of the remaining 17, 6 needed information for insurance purposes, 6 wanted to review the record for various reasons, one alleged negligence, one wanted the record sent to a school nurse, one was moving to another state, one wanted a second opinion, and one wanted her contact lens perscription. (Statistics compiled by Judy Miller, a student at Boston College Law School.)

14.   See, for example, E.G. Laforet, "The Fiction of Informed Consent," *Journal of the American Medical Association* 235 (April 12, 1976): 1579.

15.   B.R. Cassileth, et al., "Informed Consent—Why are Its Goals Imperfectly Realized?" *New England Journal of Medicine* 302, no. 16 (1980): 896.

16.   See, generally, chapter on informed consent in G.J. Annas, L.H. Glantz, and B.F. Katz, *The Rights of Doctors, Nurses and Allied Health Professionals*, (New York: Avon, 1981); and G.J. Annas, L.H. Glantz, and B.F. Katz, *Informed Consent to Human Experimentation: The Subject's Dilemma* (Cambridge, Mass.: Ballinger, 1977). And see D. Rennie, "Informed Consent by 'Well-Nigh Adject' Adults," *New England Journal of Medicine* 302, no. 16 (1980): 916. I suggest that the physician accept far more than simply the duty to improve consent forms. Physicians should accept education of the patient through the process of consent as a worthwhile therapeutic goal. To deny the possibility of informed consent is to ensure that it will never be achieved—an attitude that is immoral and illegal.

17.   L. Thomas, "On Magic in Medicine," *New England Journal of Medicine* 299 (August 31, 1978): 461, 462.

18.   M.L. Lear, *Heartsounds* (New York: Simon and Schuster, 1980), p. 47.

19.   *Ibid.*, p. 44.

20.   G.J. Annas, "The Care of Private Patients in Teaching Hospitals: Legal Implications," *Bulletin of the New York Academy of Medicine* 56, no. 4 (May 1980): 403–11.

7 MEDICAL ETHICS, THE COURTS, AND DEATH WITH DIGNITY

John J. Paris, S.J.

Case presentations at Morbidity, Mortality, and Management Conferences are a major teaching device at university hospitals. There, senior staff, residents, and interns discuss and debate medical options, decisionmaking, and value choices. A recent case presentation at a major medical center involving a 36 year old white female diabetic with chronic renal failure, retinal blindness, autonomic neuropathies, congestive heart failure, and peripheral vascular disease that required amputation of two gangrenous toes highlights some of the medical legal and ethical dilemmas confronting modern medicine.

The patient had a 20-year history of diabetes that led to the other problems, the most severe of which was her chronic kidney failure. That condition required peritoneal dialysis three times a week for the past two years. As her condition worsened, she was admitted to the hospital for a course of treatment that increased her dialysis to ten hours daily. Despite that aggressive intervention, her condition worsened and other systems failures continued.

After some two months of deterioration, the patient and her husband decided that no further aggressive or invasive measures would be considered. She refused a cardiology consultation and then requested that the dialysis be ended. All medications except insulin and analgesics were stopped; four days later the patient died.

One of the senior physicians at the conference strongly objected to the course of events. He insisted that the dialysis should have been continued. For him the "medical imperative" prevails: The physician's duty is to do everything possible to save life.

An example of that mind set is found in the accounts of the Shah of Iran's final days. As he lay dying in Cairo's Maadi Military Hospital after months of painful treatment for lymphatic cancer, his pancreas began to hemorrhage. Before blood clogged his lungs, the Shah told his doctors to avoid extraordinary measures. "I am fed up with living artificially," he said, "I don't want to die like Tito." His son, Crown Prince Reza, present at his father's bedside exclaimed, "He is dying . . . please don't let him suffer anymore."[1]

Here was a clear statement from a man who knew his condition, realized it was incurable, and understood that the advances in high technology medicine make it possible to prolong dying for weeks or even months. He wanted no part of such procedures; his family agreed. Yet after he lost four pints of blood and fell into a coma, his doctors tried unsuccessfully to revive him with electroshock treatments. Only after those attempts failed—that is, only after the Shah was dead—did the physicians remove the life-support systems.

The description recalls Ivan Illich's *Medical Nemesis*, a mad dream of progress in which we have traded our autonomy for compulsory survival in a planned and engineered hell. Life becomes only an anesthetized existence in a world turned into a hospital ward, a "managed maintenance of life on high levels of sub-lethal illness."[2] Illich argues that such a notion of "progress," in which we confidently await our aging and our cardiac resuscitations under the illusion that we are creating "health," has robbed us not only of our autonomy, but of our acceptance of the human condition—including disease, pain, and death.

With them, he adds angrily, has gone our human uniqueness, our capacity to struggle and adapt, and our ability to care for ourselves and each other. There are echoes here of Rousseau's Noble Savage: The paradise we have lost was the one within us; it was whatever enabled us, on our own, to make life feel whole and coherent, even if painful.

In an attempt to restore that sense of wholeness and to dispel if not destroy the "madness" of modern medicine "gone wild," both ethics and the law have turned their attention to the question of patients' rights to refuse medical treatment. To what extent ought that diabetic woman be able to control the course of her treatment? When if ever may she refuse life-prolonging interventions? How

many painful and debilitating occurrences did she have to undergo
before she could say "Enough!"?

VITALIST POSITION

The "vitalist" approach, which demands that everything possible be
done to save life, simplifies those questions. It requires that the parties involved abandon responsibility for difficult decisionmaking and
yield to action no matter how useless. It is a position best articulated
in *Maine Medical Center v. Baby Boy Houle*,[3] a case involving a hor-
ribly deformed newborn. His entire left side was malformed: he had
no left ear, was practically without a left eye, had a deformed left
hand; some of his vertebrae were not fused. Furthermore, he was afflicted with esophageal fistula, which prevented feeding by mouth
and allowed fluids to push up into his lungs. As his condition deteriorated, he contracted pneumonia and had several convulsive sei-
zures, which led to suspicion of severe brain damage.

The tracheal esophageal fistula, which most immediately threat-
ened the infant's life, is remediable by relatively simple surgery. The
attending physician and the boy's father wanted to forego the procedure. Several of the other physicians objected and took the case to
court. Superior Court Judge David G. Roberts's opinion forcefully
articulates the vitalist position. He stated that regardless of the newborn's condition, "At the moment of live birth there does exist a
human being entitled to the fullest protection of the law." Dismiss-
ing the attending physician's opinion that the massive deformities
and probable brain damage had rendered the life not worth saving
because it was beyond the scope of medical expertise, he ruled that
the only issue to be decided was the medical feasibility of the proposed treatment. In his view, if the corrective surgery is medically
necessary and medically feasible, it must be undertaken. And he so
ordered. (The child died shortly after the court mandated surgery.)

From Judge Roberts's perspective, courts should not consider
"quality of life" when life-saving measures are necessary. The medical and moral literature, though, evidences a more complex and
sophisticated approach to the problem. Richard McCormick, S.J., of
Georgetown University's Kennedy Center for Bioethics, has provided
the most thought-provoking analysis of the issue. In an essay in *The
Journal of the American Medical Association*, he writes that advances

in medical technology have brought us to the point where we can easily transform yesterday's medical failures into today's successes.[4] Translated into practice, this means we must shift the question from "Can we keep this patient alive?" to "What kind of life are we saving?" Such questions are irretrievably "quality of life" judgments and, McCormick argues, there is no avoiding them.

Our task, he writes, is to draw lines, develop criteria, and formulate guidelines for handling such cases, not to retreat behind talismanic incantations of "the sanctity of life" and "the worth of every individual." Such slogans, in his opinion, are the weapons of ideological battle, not the tools for analysis and enlightenment.

McCormick's own framework is developed from the traditional Judeo–Christian understanding that "It is neither human nor unchristian to say that there comes a point where an individual's condition itself represents the negation of anything truly human." When that point is reached, he asks, is not the best treatment no treatment?

There is always, of course, the lurking danger in these decisions that an individual will be valued by standards of functional utility: what the individual can do, rather than who the individual is. A sad example of that mentality occurred in the famous Johns Hopkins case in which a mongoloid child with an intestinal blockage (duodenal atresia) was allowed to starve to death over a 15-day period because his parents felt "It would be unfair to the other children to raise them with a mongoloid." James Gustafson, the University of Chicago ethicist, in a thorough and convincing criticism of that incident, argues that the presumption of life is not qualified by intelligence, nor does it yield to inconvenience.[5] There comes a point, however, when inconvenience becomes suffering and suffering becomes unbearable. At that stage, he believes, the individual no longer has an absolute moral duty of sustaining the burden.

The McCormick–Gustafson position cuts a middle ground between medical vitalism (preserving life at all costs) and medical pessimism (taking life when it seems frustrating, burdensome, or "useless"). It also aids us in a determination of how best to proceed in a case like that of the diabetic patient presented at the conference. Following their guidelines, one opts for neither a medical feasibility test nor the unreflective dismissal of treatment.

In the decisionmaking process we must begin with a determination of what is going on and the most appropriate response to that reality. In the present case, this involves an understanding of the patient's condition and the effect dialysis will have upon it. Only then is one able to make a "risk–benefit" assessment tailored to the specific needs of the individual.

This 36 year old woman had endured some twenty years of diabetic disablement and was now so debilitated that her attending physician not only held out no hope of her recovery, he had no hope for her ever leaving the hospital. The best he could offer her was a 10-hour-a-day regimen of dialysis and a prognosis of death.

"The issue," as one physician summarized it, "boils down to the quality of her life now and when she goes through the treatment." If treated, she will certainly suffer. The low probability of improvement has to be measured against that reality. Another consideration is that if the kidney failure is left untreated, she will die relatively quickly without pain or discomfort.

Those who subscribe to the proposition that "it is basic to the human condition to seek life and hold on to it however burdened" found support in much of the legal literature until the landmark Karen Ann Quinlan case forced the New Jersey Supreme Court to recognize the incredible hardships medical technology can now exact from a patient. In Quinlan we find for the first time a court ruling that "a patient cannot be forced to ensure the unendurable."[6]

ATTITUDES TOWARD DEATH

Stewart Alsop perhaps best summed up the situation in a brilliantly insightful description of his own heroic but ultimately unsuccessful fight against leukemia. "There comes a time," he writes, "when it is both wrong as well as useless to continue to resist. . . . The dying man needs to die, just as the sleepy man needs to sleep."[7] When that time comes, further expenditures of effort and expertise are not only futile, they are foolish.

At such a point, Paul Ramsey states, "We must cease doing what was once called for and begin doing what is called for now: caring for the dying."[8] That care involves comforting the dying person, not useless struggles at extending the patient's temporo-spatial existence. As Ramsey reminds us, it is the person, not the disease, who calls for our ministrations. In such circumstances the most the physician can promise is care, not a cure.

Ramsey's suggestions find reinforcement in Elizabeth Kubler-Ross's well-known studies on death and dying. These reveal that the most important problem for the dying is not death itself, but how death occurs.[9] For her, the patient's chief fear is being isolated or abandoned or being placed in a situation where people with untreatable diseases are "kept alive indefinitely by means of tubes inserted into their stomachs, or into their veins, or into their bladders, or into their rectums—victims of massive and unwarranted medical intervention upon their own particular death."[10]

In reference to a terminal cancer case, one compassionate physician has written, "It is inhuman to drag the dying patient to radiation therapy, to transfuse him repeatedly, or to give massive toxic and nauseating chemotherapy to relieve one tiny facet of an intolerable existence, thereby dragging it out for a few more agonizing days or weeks."[11] To do so to a patient who requests to die is simply an added cruelty.

One might ask how we get ourselves into such a plight. In part it is because death is perceived not as a natural function of life, but as a failure, an absolute evil, an enemy to be overcome. Thus begins the application of all available medical resources, regardless of the cost, to the patient and the patient's family. That position, of course, has always been opposed in the ethical literature where the saving of a life has not been viewed as an absolute or inflexible norm. Unfortunately, that vision is not always shared by the medical profession.

The medical and moral communities frequently do not share even a common understanding of such traditional distinctions as "ordinary/extraordinary" means of saving a life. Physicians have tended to translate "ordinary" into "customary" or what is readily available. "Extraordinary" is then understood as "heroic" or experimental treatment. With such an interpretation, the "state of the art," not the state of the patient, is the major determinant of usage. To the moralist, nonmedical features are equally dispositive and must be factored into the treatment calculus.

Paul Ramsey calls for a "reformed" medical understanding of the terms so that, depending on the condition of the patient, even the simplest and most easily applicable medication, if offering no reasonable hope of benefit to the person, is deemed "extraordinary" and thus elective.[12] Using his focus on "the person in whom the diseases inhere" and not on the disease itself, it is possible to understand why the dying patient should be treated differently from an otherwise healthy individual stricken with the same disease. For one, the treatment, painful and costly though it be, is endurable for the promise of restored health it holds; for the other, the suffering is but an added and unnecessary burden.

Ramsey's view is reinforced in the Vatican's 1980 *Declaration of Euthanasia,*[13] a document that shares his view and his unease with the traditional nomenclature. Speaking as an institution well-known for its concern for and protection of life, the Vatican writes: "Today it is very important to protect, at the moment of death, the dignity of the human person against a technological attitude that threatens to become an abuse." The text speaks of "proportionate" and "dispro-portionate" means of treatment and states that no one is obliged to employ remedies that "impose strain on the patient or suffering out of proportion to the benefits to be gained from such techniques."[14]

The document is explicit that this withholding of treatment might even include activities that have already been begun: "One cannot impose on anyone the obligation to have recourse to a technique which is already in use but which carries a risk or is burdensome." Then, in very specific language, it makes clear the fact that "such a refusal is not the equivalent of suicide." "On the contrary," it continues, echoing Illich's admonition, "it should be considered as an acceptance of the human condition."[15]

In words that speak directly to the present case, the text concludes: "When inevitable death is imminent in spite of the means used, it is permitted in conscience to take the decision to refuse forms of treatment that would only secure a precarious and burdensome prolongation of life."[16] When this is done without abandoning the patient or depriving the patient of the expected care and concern that ought to mark a professional involvement, "the doctor has no reason to reproach himself with failing to help the person in danger."[17]

Patient-centered care that focuses on the dignity of the person and not the disease allows us to recover a coherent meaning of the human condition and justifies—indeed makes obligatory—intervention against many of the invasive procedures that are possible today. We intervene because such techniques succeed not in restoring health but in robbing us of our autonomy and self-possession. They reduce us to being but a cog in some machine.

THE COURTS

Clear as the moral literature is on these issues, physicians have been reluctant to act on the basis of such consensus. Instead, following an

American tradition noted as far back as de Tocqueville, they tend to translate moral dilemmas into legal problems and turn to the courts for a definitive solution.

The first decision in this area was Karen Ann Quinlan, a case that attracted worldwide interest as everyone waited to learn if the court would, in the language of the tabloids, "pull the plug" on a 22 year old girl in a chronic vegetative condition. The New Jersey Supreme Court, in a thoughtful response to a highly sensational case, authorized the removal of a respirator that was believed to be keeping Karen Ann alive.

The Court, commenting on the "supposed imperative to sustain life at all costs," noted that physicians write "do not resuscitate" orders because they believe that in certain terminal cases " . . . it does not serve either the patient, the family, or society in any meaningful way to continue treatment."[18] In the words of one witness: "No physician that I know personally is going to try and resuscitate a man riddled with cancer and in agony and he stops breathing. They are not going to put him on a respirator . . . I think that would be the height of misuse of technology."[19]

Taking that attitude further, the Court held that if Karen Ann were "miraculously lucid for an interval" and could determine her fate, she could decide that given her condition she would not want to remain on a respirator. The Court then ruled that her guardian could make that decision in her name and it should be honored. The Court argued for such a putative decision on the grounds that such a result "should be accepted by a society the overwhelming majority of whose members would, we think, in similar circumstances, exercise such a choice in the same way for themselves or for those closest to them."[20]

To buttress its position, the *Quinlan* Court employed several of the principles regularly used by the ethicists: the distinction between so-called active and passive euthanasia (i.e., "self-infliction of deadly harm and a self-determination against artificial life support in the face of irreversible, painful and certain imminent death"); the humane decision against resuscitive or maintenance therapy for terminally ill patients; and the distinction between curing the ill and comforting and easing the dying. The Court offered, "We think these attitudes represent a balanced implementation of a profoundly realistic perspective on the meaning of life and death and that they respect the whole Judeo–Christian tradition of regard for human life."[21]

The Court reiterated Ramsey's position that "one would have to think that the use of the same respirator or like support could be considered 'ordinary' in the context of the possibly curable patient but 'extraordinary' in the context of . . . an irreversibly doomed patient."[22] It then authorized the guardian to have Karen Ann's respirator discontinued, even though it was thought that such an action would result in her death. (For the tragic story of how the physician in that case thwarted the will of the Court and the parents and continued Karen Ann on the respirator for six weeks until she could be successfully weaned from it, see Joseph Quinlan, *Karen Ann*.[23] Some four years later Karen Ann is still alive and still in a chronic vegetative state).

SAIKEWICZ CASE

The following year an equally difficult medical case was brought before the Massachusetts courts. Joseph Saikewicz, a profoundly retarded 67 year old, became ill with acute myelogenous leukemia, an invariably fatal disease that, though noncurable, may in some instances be slowed by chemotherapy. His physician and the Belchertown State School authorities where he had resided for nearly 50 years had to determine the proper treatment. The physicians stressed, and the Probate Court accepted the arguments, that it was not in the best interests of the patient to undergo chemotherapy. The treatments would offer a 30 percent chance of a remission of some two–thirteen months, but would produce serious side effects that Saikewicz would experience but not comprehend.

In a thorough and insightful opinion, the Supreme Judicial Court (SJC) provided an exceptionally fine substantive statement on the issue, one that carefully laid out the current state of medical ethics.[24] The Court chose to focus on three issues: the right of any person, competent or incompetent, to decline life-prolonging treatment; the legal standard for noncompetents; and the procedure to be followed in arriving at such a decision.

Interestingly, the opinion began with the admission that existing legal doctrine was unable to resolve the novel issues raised in the case. The SJC, admitting that the law necessarily lags behind the most advanced thinking in every area, turned to the reflections of health care, theology, moral ethics, and philosophy for guidance and insight on how to deal with terminally ill patients. From these it noted several shifts in the medical approach to such patients. For example, it noted that prior to the development of advances in technology, the physician tended to perceive his or her duty as that of making every conceivable effort to prolong life. That was true in part because the physician had a very limited ability to ward off or postpone death. With the development of new techniques, serious questions arise as to the wisdom of such a policy.

One response to that changing reality is that "physicians have begun to realize that in many cases the effect of using extraordinary measures to prolong life is to only prolong suffering, isolate the family from their loved one at a time when they may be close at hand or result in economic ruin of the family."[25]

In the conclusion of its analysis the SJC wrote:

> The current state medical ethics in this area is expressed by one commentator who states that: "We should not use extraordinary means of prolonging life or its semblance when, after careful consideration, consultation and the application of the most well conceived therapy it becomes apparent that there is no hope of recovery of the patient. Recovery should not be defined simply as the ability to remain alive; it should mean life without intolerable suffering." Lewis, "Machine Medicine and Its Relation to the Fatally Ill," 206 *J.A.M.A.* 387 (1968).
>
> Our decision in this case is consistent with the current medical ethos in this area.[26]

Further, the SJC concurred with the Quinlan decision in adopting the Ramsey/Kubler–Ross thesis that we can and ought to distinguish between "curing the ill and comforting and easing the dying." It accepted the stand that physicians ought not treat the hopeless and dying as if they were curable. Rather, in the Court's view, they ought to recognize that the dying are more in need of comfort than of treatment.

These positions, undergirded by recent developments in the law on informed consent and respect for the right of privacy, were the basis for the Court's authorization of the withholding of chemotherapy for Saikewicz. The Court acknowledged the state's interest in preserving life, but where that preservation is tendentious at best and attained only at traumatic cost, the SJC recognized the right of an individual to forego that cost.

In an interesting turn of the argument, the Court reversed the thesis that the value of life is lessened or cheapened by a decision to refuse treatment. It ruled that the value of life is diminished by the failure to allow a competent human being the right of choice and the right of privacy, that is, the right to be left alone.

The more difficult problem is the attribution of these rights to the incompetent. As was seen earlier, there are those who argue strenuously that the physician must always provide treatment to the incompetent or risk devaluing their dignity and worth. The SJC rejected that proposition and in a precedent-shattering contribution to the developing trend in the law, ruled that "the principles of equality and respect for all individuals require that a choice exist for incompetents as well as competents."[27] To do otherwise," it stated, "would be to treat wards of the state as a person of lesser status or dignity than others."

Having recognized the right of an incompetent to refuse life-prolonging treatment, the Court was faced with the awesome task (in a case of first impression) of framing an adequate rationale to explain how that right might be exercised. It did so with an interesting yoking of the long-standing legal doctrine of substituted judgment with a Rawlsian reconstruction of the mental world of a "rational" incompetent.

Substituted judgment, a doctrine first articulated in English law over 150 years ago,[28] deals with authorization of gifts from the estate of incompetents. The English court reasoned this could be done by "donning the mental mantle of the incompetent," that is, what we might reasonably conclude the individual would do if the individual could understand the present situation.

That theory of respect for the integrity and autonomy of all persons found renewed vigor in John Rawls's highly influential *A Theory of Justice*, where he argued that maintaining the integrity of the person means that we act toward the person "as we have reason to believe he would choose for himself if he were capable of reasoning and deciding rationally."[29] This does not mean that we can impute preferences to the person that were never held. But, as is true in the case of Saikewicz, where no preferences have been made, our task is to ask how we would act for ourselves if we were in a similar position.

Applying the substituted judgment theory to Saikewicz, the SJC concluded that the Probate Court, the physicians, and the school staff all operated in the best interests of Joseph Saikewicz; they chose what appeared to be the least detrimental alternative available for the patient. It also observed that none of the parties used "quality of life" judgments as a value of the patient's life, and that great care was taken to respect the worth of Saikewicz's life precisely because of his vulnerable status.

The Court was particularly careful in its fashioning of the "quality of life" statements to dispel any possible interpretation that the low quality of life of a mentally retarded individual was a determining factor in this case. It announced its regret that "the vague and perhaps ill-chosen term" had crept into the testimony. It also made explicit its understanding that the phrase as used referred to "the continuing state of pain and disorientation precipitated by the chemotherapy treatment" and not to a "value of life" judgment.[30]

The third item of the SJC's concern, the procedure by which decisions to withhold life-prolonging treatment for noncompetents are to be made, is of great interest to both the legal-medical community and to the public at large. It is also, perhaps, the least satisfactory and most controversial section of the opinion.

The Court mandated that in questions of providing or withholding life-prolonging treatment from all alleged incompetents (not only state wards), a probate court determination of competency must be made. If the individual is adjudged incompetent, a guardian ad litem must be appointed who will represent the patient at a full adversarial hearing and who must defend the proposition that the treatment should be administered. The Court requires this procedure so that "all viewpoints and alternatives will be aggressively pursued and examined."

The effect of this ruling is to add full adversarial hearings with competing witnesses, opposing counsel, and the trauma of courtroom drama to the already stressful decisionmaking process involved in the withholding of treatment from the terminally ill noncompetent patient. At the practical level, then, every time a patient suffering from a terminal illness lapses into disorientation, senility, or unconsciousness, the family and physicians will be plunged into the unwelcome, cumbersome, and costly arena of litigation if they determine that further treatment is unwarranted. The predictable result will be the unnecessary continuation of the treatment by the physician, and suffering for the patient and his family.

The New Jersey Supreme Court foresaw that result in the Quinlan case and sought to obviate it by locating the decisionmaking mechanism within the guardian–family–physician group, subject in difficult or novel cases to ratification by a hospital ethics committee. It did so because it believed decisions on "the nature, extent, and duration of care" are primarily the physician's responsibility. Shifting that role to the court was judged to be "a gratuitous encroachment upon the medical profession's field of competence."[31] It would also prove to be a time-consuming and cumbersome process that would overburden already clogged courts.

The Massachusetts bench feared no such results. In very specific terms it declared: "We reject the approach adopted by the New Jersey Supreme Court." In doing so, it appropriated to the courts the role of making all life and death decisions for every incompetent in the Commonwealth. It did this because, in its phrasing, "that responsibility is not to be entrusted to any other group purporting to represent the 'mortality and conscience of our society,' no matter how highly motivated or impressively constituted."[32]

SPRING CASE

Criticizing the approach of the Massachusetts bench in the Saikewicz case, Richard McCormick and André Helligers of Georgetown's Kennedy Institute of Ethics wrote: "Much that is at best inappropriate, at worse abusive, could happen to a patient as the adversary procedures unfold. The result is that patients are now to suffer, often needlessly, for the purposes of the court's procedures."[33] That is precisely what happened in the case of Earle Spring, a 78 year old senile man whose wife and son sought to stop the hemodialysis treatments that he had undergone for over a year.

Both his family and physician believed the treatment offered the terminally ill Spring no substantial benefit. It promised no improvement of his underlying disease. But much like the Shah of Iran's case, there was the possibility of extending his suffering. Further, the family and physician believed that their request was what Earle Spring would have wanted. They acted only to meet his desires and his "best interests" and did so within the normative guidelines of medical ethics and respect for patients' rights.

Since the family resided in Massachusetts, they followed the procedures for the cessation of treatment of terminally ill incompetent patients outlined in *Saikewicz*. The Probate Court, adhering to those procedures, appointed a guardian ad litem to represent Earle Spring, conducted an adversary hearing, and issued an order to terminate the treatment.

At this stage one would anticipate nothing more need be done. There was no dramatic "plug to pull," no disagreement among the

family, no doubt of the motive, no dispute over the treatment protocol. All that remained were the prayers of a dedicated, close-knit
family gathered at the bedside of a dying father. But the guardian ad
litem objected. Despite the *Saikewicz* ruling to the contrary, he insisted that there had to be some positive evidence of Spring's will
and not merely a "substituted judgment" before a Court could order
the termination of treatment.

That maneuver was carried through Probate, Appeals, and Supreme Court hearings until finally, some fourteen months after the
initial hearing, while still receiving the Court ordered treatments,
Earle Spring's heart gave out. In a posthumous opinion on the case
the SJC stated, "The [Probate] judge's findings were not clearly
erroneous and the judge's [original] order was in accordance with
law."[34] The original family–physician request should have been
honored, but for the purposes of court-mandated procedures Earle
Spring suffered an additional year of hemodialysis. His family experienced that suffering, while enduring the pain and cost of litigation, near financial ruin, banner headlines, television reporting, and
the agony of a public dying.

FOX CASE

A similar sad tale is told in the recent judicial intervention involving
a termination of treatment controversy, the case of Brother Joseph
Fox. Fox, an 83 year old religious brother, had entered Nassau Hospital for a routine hernia operation. During the course of the surgery
he suffered cardiorespiratory arrest, and when resuscitated was found
to be in a chronic vegetative condition. Since Brother Fox had agreed
with the Catholic Church's teachings that heroic measures to prolong
life were unnecessary, had discussed those issues in conversations
about the Quinlan case, and had clearly stated he did not want any
"extraordinary" measures taken to prolong his own life, his guardian, Father Eichner, asked the physicians to remove the respirator
which was keeping him alive. They refused. The surgeon, Dr. Edward
Kelly, asserted that once such a medical procedure was started, "it
should not be withdrawn." A spokesman for the hospital reinforced
his stand when he stated, "Our mission is to do all that we can to
maintain life."[35]

Father Eichner then sought a court order to have the respirator
removed. The trial court so ordered, and in words that ought to be

underscored and capitalized, addressed itself to the physicians' fears
that once they have started a respirator "medically and legally they
would not dare shut it off." "It is important," said the court, "that
the law not create a disincentive to the fullest treatment of patients
by making it impossible for them in at least some extreme circumstances to choose to end treatment which has proven unsuccessful."[36] With that standard, the trial court provided legal support
for Paul Ramsey's well-known position that, in fact, there is more
moral warrant for turning off a machine than for never having started
it; that is, once the patient has been given the benefit of all known
procedures and these prove unsuccessful in restoring health, they
need not be uselessly continued. It is to be hoped that the legal recognition of that moral reality will help overcome physician timidity
in similar cases.

The District Attorney appealed the trial court's decision, but in a
unanimous opinion the Appellate Division of the New York State
Supreme Court agreed with the original ruling. As in *Saikewicz*, the
Appellate Court acknowledged "the right of the terminally ill to refuse treatment and to allow the natural process of death to run its
course."[37] It also agreed that this right accrued to the competent
and incompetent alike.

Unfortunately, the procedural aspects of the *Fox* case are even
more troubling than those in *Saikewicz*. After asserting that these
rights applied to all terminally ill patients, the Appellate Division substantially restricted the termination of extraordinary life-supporting
treatments in incompetent patients in two very substantial ways. For
reasons the Court believed were "self-apparent," it established very
restrictive medical criteria for the activation of the patient's right to
terminate treatment: only those terminally ill who are in a permanent vegetative coma with extremely remote probability of regain-
ing cognitive brain function qualify. This stringent standard covers a
dramatic, but small fraction of terminally ill incompetent patients.
What of the rights of the others? Under this ruling, for example,
Earle Spring would have no claim for relief. Nor would Joseph Saikewicz, whose case provided most of the legal support for the *Fox*
opinion.

A clue to the Court's motive is found in its rationale for termination of life-prolonging treatments in the chronic vegetative patient:

As a matter of established fact such a patient has no health and, in the true
sense, no life, for the State to protect. . . . Indeed, with Roe [abortion deci-

sion] in mind, it is appropriate to note that the State's interest in preservation of the life of the fetus would appear greater than any possible interest
the State may have in maintaining continued life of a terminally ill comatose
patient . . . [whose] claim to personhood is certainly no greater than that of
a fetus.

In essence, the Appellate Division asserts that its concern for the
"sanctity of life" is maintained because the chronic vegetative patient is, in fact, dead. Or, if not dead, certainly deserving no more
state interest than does the fetus. The potential abuses implicit in
such an approach to the comotose patient are staggering.

Having set such a dangerous course, the Appellate Division was
quick to insist that such awesome decisions "must reside with the
judicial process and the judicial process alone." In doing so, it rejected the *Quinlan* standard. Instead, it adopted the approach and
the language of *Saikewicz* on the requirement of court involvement.

The *Fox* court intensified the requirements for treatment termination by stipulating that the following provisions be applied "in
each case on an individual patient-to-patient basis":

1. A physician certifies that the patient is terminally ill and in an
    irreversible, permanent vegetative coma, and that prospects for
    recovery of cognitive brain functions are extremely remote.
2. The case is then presented to a hospital committee of at least
    three physicians, for confirmation of diagnosis.
3. If the medical judgment is thus confirmed, judicial proceedings
    must then be instituted for permission to withdraw life-sustain-
    ing measures.
4. The attorney general and district attorney are notified and may
    select additional physicians to examine the patient.
5. A guardian ad litem is appointed to protect the patient's inter-
    ests.
6. A court hearing is held.
7. The court determines that the prognosis is correct.
8. The court issues an order to discontinue the extraordinary treat-
    ment.

In sum, a minimum of four to six physicians, five attorneys, and
one judge are now required to determine an outcome that traditional ethical analysis—and the Appellate Division itself—recognized
as belonging to every patient: the right to decline extraordinary
treatment.

The New York court believed that such procedures are necessary to protect the rights of the incompetent and to mitigate a difficult ethical problem facing the medical profession. It also believed that, ultimately, the procedures affirm the dignity and worth of human life. For Brother Fox, this decision meant five months of chronically vegetative existence in an intensive-care unit, an $87,000 hospital bill, and $20,000 in legal fees. If his heart had not failed in the course of the legal dispute, the expenses might still be mounting, since the legal contest continued in a higher court, the New York Court of Appeals.

The District Attorney again appealed, and on review the Court of Appeals voided all of the substantive and procedural rulings of the lower court except for the specific authorization of the termination of treatment.[38] Rather than follow the right of privacy and substituted judgment argument, New York's highest court used the common law right of every person "of adult years and sound mind . . . to determine what shall be done with his own body" as the basis for its opinion in support of Brother Fox's right to decline treatment. Then, in a very restricted ruling, the Court decreed that such decisions could be made for incompetents only when there is no hope of recovery and where there is "clear and convincing" evidence that the patient had left instructions to end life-sustaining procedures in such circumstances. To reinforce its position, the Court made it clear that "this standard forbids relief whenever the evidence is loose, equivocal or contradictory," or if it emanates from "causal remarks made at some social gathering" or those made by one "too young to realize or feel the consequences of his statements."[39]

The Court very appropriately wanted to protect children and other incompetents from those who would deny them life-sustaining medical treatment for reasons other than the patients' best interests. But it failed to understand that for a Joseph Saikewicz or an Earle Spring, such treatment only prolongs suffering and dying. In so ruling, the New York Court abrogated the fundamental right recognized in the Vatican's *Declaration*: that all humans—competent or incompetent, articulate or uninformed—may decline extraordinary means of prolonging life when it becomes apparent that there is no hope of recovery.

CONCLUSION

The only option open for families of those not covered by the *Eichner* standard is to seek a legislative change or to "apply to courts for a ruling on the propriety of conduct which might seriously affect their charges." The result of such an approach is, in the words of Father Eichner, "a lawyer's paradise, not to mention a doctor's bonanza." "It may be fine law," he states, "but it is certainly not true justice."[40] For who can afford all these doctors and lawyers, or endure the additional trauma of court procedures? And why is it all necessary?

For some, there is a lurking fear that an unscrupulous doctor or a selfish son or daughter would "do in" a little old grandmother before her time. But if we try to set up guidelines to make the medical profession 100 percent ethical and to make families sin-free, we run the risk of creating greater evil. As the history of social organization well documents, attempts to legislate a perfect society wind up with a greater universal harm.

John Rawls's *Theory of Justice* provides the essential insight into how we might proceed in such cases. He proposes a theory of "justice as fairness," in which what ought to be done is determined by asking: "What would we agree to if operating behind a 'veil of ignorance' we did not know what role we would play in life: rich/poor, doctor/patient, judge/terminally ill person sustained by life-support apparatus?" What a person would agree to for each position, not knowing one's own role, Rawls asserts, is the fundamental minimal demand of justice. What indeed would one want if one were Earle Spring, Joseph Fox, or a 36 year old diabetic suffering from multiple failures and forced to endure ten hours a day of dialysis to maintain existence? I suspect that one would insist on a procedure that would not be unreasonably dragged out, that would not distress one's family, and that—as much as the human condition of fallibility allows—would not fail to safeguard the right to decide whether to struggle for yet another morning or slip gently into the night.

Death is a personal matter, one that as in the case presentation is most aptly acceded to by the actual patient or for the incompetent patient by those who, in the *Fox* court's words, "knew and loved the patient personally." Technical developments may have made the issue more dramatic, but the questions of life and death and of who should decide are not new; they have been debated since the dawn of history.

A fortunate by-product of the recent court opinions is a renewed interest in and awareness of patients' rights to refuse medications or treatments that do not offer substantial hope or benefit. The woman in the above case understood that principle, as did her physician, and so her suffering was not needlessly extended. Furthermore, all involved understood that unanimity of patient–family–physician opinion, when that opinion conforms to professional standards, has traditionally been and ought to be the norm for a decision not to treat. Without evidence of malevolent motives or medical negligence, there is no need for judicial intervention. As Chief Justice Warren Burger once observed of such life and death decisions, "They are among the myriads of problems and troubles which judges are powerless to solve; and that is as it should be."[41] The King, broken and defeated, is dying. There is a call for a physician. Kent cries:

> Vex not his ghost: O, let him pass! He hates him much that would upon the rack of this tough world stretch him out longer.
>
> —*King Lear*

NOTES TO CHAPTER 7

1. *Newsweek*, August 11, 1980, p. 38.
2. Ivan Illich, *Medical Nemesis* (New York: Bantam Books, 1976), p. 25.
3. Maine Medical Center v. Houle, Superior Court, Cumberland. Docket No. 74–145, February 14, 1974.
4. Richard A. McCormick, "To Save or Let Die: The Dilemma of Modern Medicine," *Journal of the American Association* 229 (1974): 172.
5. James Gustafson, "Mongolism, Parental Desires and the Right to Life," *Perspectives in Biology and Medicine* 16 (1972–73): 529.
6. *In re* Karen Ann Quinlan, 70 New Jersey 10; 355 A. 2d 647, 663 (1976).
7. Stewart Alsop, *Stay of Execution* (Philadelphia: J.B. Lippincott, 1973), p. 271.
8. Paul Ramsey, "On (Only) Caring for the Dying," in *The Patient as Person* (New Haven: Yale University Press, 1970), p. 159.
9. Elizabeth Kubler–Ross, *On Death and Dying* (New York: Macmillan Co., 1969).
10. E.H. Rynearson, "You are Standing at Bedside of a Patient Dying of Untreatable Cancer," *CA* 9 (May–June, 1954): 84.
11. J. Engelbert Dunphy, "On Caring for the Patient with Cancer," *Bulletin of the American College of Surgeons* 61 (October 1976): 12.

12. Paul Ramsey, *The Patient as Person*, pp. 126–27.
13. Sacred Congregation for the Doctrine of the Faith, *Declaration on Euthanasia* (Vatican City, 1980).
14. *Ibid.*, p. 11.
15. *Ibid.*
16. *Ibid.*
17. *Ibid.*
18. *In re* Karen Ann Quinlan, 70 New Jersey 10; 355 A.2d 647, 660 (1976).
19. Julius Korein, M.D., *In re* Quinlan, 70 New Jersey 10; 355 A.2d 647, 660 (1976).
20. 355 A.2d at 664.
21. 355 A.2d at 667.
22. 355 A.2d at 668.
23. Joseph Quinlan, *Karen Ann* (New York: Doubleday, 1977).
24. Paul Ramsey, *The Patient as Person*, pp. 126–127.
25. 370 N.E.2d at 423.
26. 370 N.E.2d at 424.
27. 370 N.E.2d at 427–28.
28. Exparte Whitebread, *in re* Hinde, a Lunatic, Eng. Rep. Vol. 35, (1816), at 878.
29. John Rawls, *A Theory of Justice* (Cambridge, Mass.: Harvard University Press, 1971).
30. 370 N.E.2d at 432.
31. 355 A.2d at 669.
32. 370 N.E.2d at 435.
33. Richard McCormick and André Helligers, "The Spector of Joseph Saikewicz: Mental Incompetence and the Law," *America* 138 (1978): 257.
34. *In re* Spring, Mass., 405 N.E.2d 115, 123 (1978).
35. John J. Paris, "Court Intervention and the Diminution of Patients' Rights: The Case of Brother Joseph Fox," *New England Journal of Medicine* 303 (1980): 876.
36. In the matter of Eichner, Supreme Court, Nassau County, No. 21242–I/79, December 6, 1979 at 29.
37. *In re* Eichner, AD2d, 637 E, March 28, 1980, Supreme Court: Appellate Division, Second Department, at 62–63.
38. Eichner v. Dillon, New York Court of Appeals, No. 658, March 31, 1981.
39. Eichner v. Dillon, March 31, 1981 at 13.
40. Paris, "Court Intervention," *supra* note 35 at 877.
41. Application of President and Directors of Georgetown College, Inc., 331 F.2d 1010, 1017 (D.C. Cir. 1964), Burger, J. dissenting).

8 THE GERIATRIC PATIENT
Ethical Issues in Care and Treatment

Ruth Macklin

In any discussion about medical ethics, it is always fair to ask whether the ethical issues that arise in a particular setting or regarding a particular patient population are unique to that setting or population, or whether the same ethical concerns mark the care of patients in other facilities or from other special groups. It would be an easy, if not rather boring, exercise if we could simply transfer the moral problems and any proposed solutions to them from one setting, or one patient population, to another. Yet it would be surprising if there were no common ethical problems among different areas of medical practice. After all, medical treatment and research, nursing services, administration of health care facilities, and other activities in the sphere of medical and health care all focus on the patient: ill, ailing, or injured people. With regard to geriatric patients, these questions need reply: Are there special ethical problems that arise in caring for elderly patients, problems that never or rarely occur in general medicine or with other special populations? Are there special ethical problems that arise in caring for such patients in an extended care facility, problems that never or rarely exist in the context of ambulatory care or short-term medical facilities?

It should come as no surprise to learn that the answers to these questions are both "yes" and "no." Similarities and differences between the situations that give rise to ethical issues in the care and treatment of geriatric patients can be found elsewhere in medicine. It is only very recently, with the rise of the medical specialty of geriatrics, that medically related ethical problems of the elderly as a special patient population have begun to receive attention. Like the typical adult patient, many elderly persons are perfectly capable of granting (or refusing) consent for medical treatment, and of making life choices following their release from the hospital. Like other special populations, most notably mental patients, those elderly who suffer from senile dementia lack the capacity to grant informed consent or to participate in decisionmaking regarding their care and treatment.

Yet in spite of these evident similarities, the elderly differ in a number of relevant respects from other patient populations. Elderly patients as they near the end of the life span, often have a different set of values in their assessments of the quality of life than do younger persons. Furthermore, elderly persons who have begun to decline in their mental capacity nevertheless have a lifetime of experiences and accomplishments that inform their wants and perceived needs relating to medical treatment and aftercare. Since there is no expectation that they will reenter the work force, or enjoy a return to productivity, their plight differs significantly from that of other hospitalized adults who are better able to exercise their autonomy as patients. Finally, like all residents of extended care facilities, the elderly in such settings are at risk for increased dependency and other typical consequences of institutionalization.

Key concepts in bioethics include paternalism, autonomy, and informed consent. These assume special importance in the care and treatment of geriatric patients because of the prevalence of dementing illness. When elderly persons suffer slight cognitive impairment, to what extent should they be permitted (or encouraged) to make decisions regarding their own medical care and treatment, as well as other life choices? Under what conditions is it justifiable to remove from people their decisionmaking autonomy about matters affecting primarily themselves, when they have enjoyed a lifetime of such autonomy? Should a finding of incompetence in one area automatically be transferred to or assumed to exist in, any other area? (Compare competency to manage one's financial affairs, competency to make a will, and competency to grant or refuse consent for a medical procedure.) Are the considerations that might support some form of paternalism (coercing people for their own good) the same for all special populations whose competency may be in doubt, or do special considerations obtain in the case of the elderly? When elderly persons of questionable capacity disagree with what others think is best for them regarding a medical or life choice decision, how should such differences be handled? What role should other family members play in the settlement of such disagreements? This last question is of crucial importance for geriatric patients, since if they have not been declared *legally* incompetent, family members are not automatically empowered to override their relative's medical decision (for example, a refusal of amputation).

According to one recent account, "estimates are that approximately 10% of persons older than 65 years have clinically important intellectual impairment. In a survey of nursing homes published in 1978, respondents to a questionnaire reported that 50% to 75% of the residents in their facilities were intellectually impaired."[1] Another set of figures reports that "one out of every six persons over the age of 65—about 1½ million people—is at least moderately demented. Sixty to eighty percent of nursing home patients are demented."[2] These figures are roughly the same, and they suggest that the problem of senile dementia is one of considerable magnitude.

The magnitude of the problem is only one dimension that gives rise to ethical concerns. Another is the uncertainty and variability of judgments about the mental status of elderly patients. Several factors contribute to the uncertainty and variability of such judgments, and at the risk of repeating what is well known, it is worth citing a number of those factors to illustrate the complexity of the problem of making judgments of competence.

The first factor is the reversibility or irreversibility of impaired intellectual function. Obviously, it is important to assess the causes of mental impairment whenever possible, whether or not there exist clear or uncontroversial criteria for determining what a person should be permitted to do or to decide at a particular level of competence. The fact that we lack such criteria points to still another problem, to be addressed shortly. It seems clear that if impaired mental functioning can be reversed, not only should efforts be made to reverse it, but also that an ethical requirement in such situations is that any decisions about life choices affecting the elderly should be postponed if possible until mental function is restored. Although these points may seem obvious, it remains true that demands on the time and resources of personnel in a hospital or extended care facility often prevent prompt or accurate diagnoses, especially in an area of emerging medical knowledge, such as the causes of dementia. Since these causes are numerous, and include everything from depression to deficiencies in nutrients, prompt and thorough diagnostic workups are vital for the prospects of reversing mental impairment.

A fact that bears directly on the broader ethical issues in treating geriatric patients in an extended care facility is that the most common causes of *reversible* impaired intellectual function are therapeutic drug intoxication, depression, and metabolic or infectious disorders.[3] This fact suggests that adequate knowledge on the part of physicians and other health care workers, and the devotion of sufficient time and effort to make timely and accurate diagnoses, can go a long way toward reversing this unfortunate condition in many elderly patients. Especially troubling are the facts about the adverse effects of medication. "An enormous number of drugs have been implicated, including diuretics, digitalis, oral antidiabetic drugs, analgesics, anti-inflammatory agents, sedatives, and psychopharmacologic agents."[4] Add to the sheer number of drugs having this effect the further consideration that the elderly metabolize drugs differently from younger persons and that they are often being treated with multiple drugs, leading to toxicity from drug interactions, and it is not hard to conclude that a significant cause of mental impairment in elderly patients is iatrogenic.

More problematic from another standpoint are the disorders that cause *irreversible* dementia. According to a report of the National Institute on Aging Task Force, two of them—Alzheimer's disease and multi-infarct dementia—account for approximately 80 percent of the dementias of old age.[5] Unlike the reversible causes of mental impairment, which must be diagnosed and treated promptly, but in which actions or decisions on the part of the elderly can often await their improvement, cases of irreversible mental decline pose a different set of problems. A poignant moral dilemma in such cases is when, how much, and in what manner to disclose to a patient the prognosis of the disease and the facts about impending decline. We need to develop a sensitive and humane approach both to informing Alzheimer's patients of the details and prognosis of their disease, and to working with families in preparing for the patient's decline in mental capacity—a decline that has both short-term and long-term implications for decisions and actions concerning legal, financial, and other life circumstances. The ethical questions surrounding disclosure are linked with the more general issue of paternalism toward elderly persons who are in physical and mental decline, and whose growing dependence on others demands a morally sound approach.

Another factor lending complexity to the problem of making judgments of competency in the elderly is the existence of several different tests of competency—tests that may yield conflicting results when applied to elderly persons suffering from dementia. The above-noted report mentions several tests commonly used in the mental status examination: orientation for time, place, and persons; short-term memory, arithmetic calculation; ability to name objects; comprehension of spoken and written language; ability to write a spontaneous sentence; and ability to copy simple geometric figures. The report asserts that the impression of progressively deteriorating mental function can be confirmed and documented by such tests, but that assertion may be misleading. Even if these commonly used tests succeed in confirming a supposition that a patient is undergoing progressive mental decline, they yield no clear picture of the tasks or judgments that the patient is able or unable to perform beyond those specifically measured in the tests themselves. What does a test for a patient's ability to do arithmetic calculations have to do with that patient's understanding of a proposed medical procedure for which the patient's consent is sought? What does an inability to copy simple geometric figures tell us about a person's ability to make changes in his or her will? One problematic example is that of an elderly patient suffering from senile dementia who exhibits severe impairment of short-term memory, yet scores 110 on a standard psychometric instrument for measuring IQ. When two different tests of competency yield conflicting results, which one should be selected as a measure of the patient's competency? Or do they not conflict at all because they measure discrete capacities?

The exitence of multiple measures for evaluating competency is one consideration contributing to the complexity of this issue. A related but quite different issue is the value question of how strong or how weak tests of competency should be—a factor that bears directly on the ethics of paternalistic treatment of elderly persons of questionable capacity. Since these conceptual and ethical issues surrounding judgments of competency are directly related to a patient's ability to grant or refuse consent for a wide variety of biomedical interventions, as well as to engage in a number of different life tasks, it is important to look carefully at current practices and knowledge in related fields. Recent research has concentrated largely on psychiatric patients in an attempt to gain a better understanding of competency as it relates to various tasks. The trend in both law and medicine in the last few years has been toward developing a notion of variable competence, and toward selecting situation-specific criteria for judging competence, rather than viewing it as a global attribute of people.

In a recent article discussing currently used tests of competency to consent to treatment, the authors describe five basic categories into which such tests fall.[6] These are: (1) evidencing a choice; (2) "reasonable" outcome of choice; (3) choice based on "rational" reasons; (4) ability to understand; and (5) actual understanding. Noting that these categories overlap, the authors point out that the tests range from the weakest test of competency to the strongest, with the tests at the lowest level being most respectful of the autonomy of patient decisionmaking. Just which of these tests ought to be used to determine the competence of elderly patients is a question not easy to answer, and one that probably would elicit some controversy among caregivers, family members, and elderly patients themselves. These same authors argue that

> the test that is actually applied combines elements of all of the tests described above. However, the circumstances in which competency becomes an issue determine which elements of which tests are stressed and which are underplayed. Although in theory competency is an independent variable that determines whether or not the patient's decision to accept or refuse treatment is to be honored, in practice it seems to be dependent on the interplay of two other variables, and risk/benefit ratio of treatment and the valence of the patient's decision, i.e., whether he or she consents to or refuses treatment.[7]

Since questions of individual preference and personal values are often bound up in treatment refusals, it is crucial to try to assess the reasons behind an elderly person's refusal to consent. The stricter the standard of competence, in the interest of protecting patients from their own unwise decisions, the more autonomy is traded for a gain in benevolent paternalism. It is generally assumed that when elderly patients suffer diminished capacity, and thus cannot speak on their own behalf, caregivers and family have their "best interests" at heart and will act in accordance with those interests; yet the validity of this and related assumptions has yet to be adequately explored. The question of where the presumption ought to lie regarding elderly persons of questionable competence is more a matter for decision than a matter of scientific discovery of the precise attributes that constitute competency. Should the presumption lie in their ability to judge and decide for themselves, suggesting the adoption of a weak test of competency? Or should the presumption lie on the side of impaired ability to judge, suggesting the adoption of a strong test of competency? We seek to avoid erring in either of two opposite directions: being too paternalistic with the elderly, taking their dependency and "childlike" attributes as grounds for coercing them for their own good; and on the other hand, being too permissive in respecting their autonomy, thereby opening the door to self-destructive or other irresponsible acts. The one evil consists of violating the cherished value of individual freedom; the other evil is to allow harm, destruction, or even death to befall a helpless, dependent person with declining mental and physical faculties.

These ethical dilemmas point to a research agenda for studying problems of competency and informed consent in the elderly. For elderly persons of doubtful or declining competence, the following problem areas deserve further study. Current practices surrounding disclosure by physicians, other health care workers, and family members to elderly patients with declining mental functioning need to be analyzed, focusing on the values to be attained by adhering to any particular policy or practice. What are the conditions under which full and frank disclosure about a patient's condition should take place? Are there special circumstances under which information should be withheld? How can such patients be helped to prepare themselves, psychologically and emotionally, for a deterioration in their cognitive capacities? What supports can be offered to the families of patients such as those suffering from Alzheimer's disease, especially in regard to assessing the appropriate time and method of disclosure?

Further work is also called for concerning the problem of paternalism toward the elderly who suffer from growing incompetence, and of the autonomy of aging individuals to make decisions and perform tasks both related and unrelated to biomedical procedures. Where ought the presumption lie: with the elderly themselves, to demonstrate their continued competence? Or with those who challenge their competence, to show that the principle of beneficence dictates treating those with senile dementia as incompetent, and therefore no longer autonomous, agents? There is a special poignancy to the problem of the growing incompetence of elderly persons, stemming from their own awareness of that decline, and the fact that having once been normally functioning adults, they are witness to their own mental and physical deterioration and to changes in the attitudes and behavior of others toward them. Even in cases where mental functioning is clearly impaired, a morally sound approach dictates enlisting the participation of elderly patients as much as possible in decisions regarding their own care and treatment.

At the outset I mentioned the prospect of special ethical problems that arise in caring for patients in an extended care facility. Although the characteristics of "total institutions"—to use Erving Goffman's term—are by now well-known, it is worth repeating here that especially in the case of elderly persons, residents of such facilities often respond to their environment in ways that exacerbate their already declining capacities. One writer describes the situation as follows:

> Many nursing homes, geriatric wards, and mental hospitals have the characteristics of total institutions: simply by their institutional structures and expectations, they determine the behavior of their residents. . . . According to one description (Citrin and Dixon, 1977), a radical alteration in life-style following institutionalization, joined with increasing demands by the institution's staff and decreasing physical functioning frequently brings about socially withdrawn, confused, or disoriented behavior among the elderly. Thus (Butler 1975), substantial numbers of patients in mental hospitals develop a chronic state of psychological dependence and deterioration. Infantilization and loss of self-image are frequently the result of institutionalization and interaction with the institution's staff. . . .[8]

The term "infantilization" is a key one here, and serves as a reminder that the elderly in decline are not, of course, literally "infants," in spite of many behavioral similarities. The ethical problem is to determine to what extent care and treatment of the elderly who exhibit "infantile behavior" in the metaphorical sense should be treated as we deem it proper to treat infants and small children—that is, in accordance with a justifiable pattern of paternalistic control. Insofar as the institutional structure of an extended care facility deepens those problems by reinforcing the dependency and childlike behavior of its residents, it seems possible—at least in principle—to make changes in that structure, and thereby lessen the ethical problems to some extend. Let me illustrate.

I recently learned of the existence of several nursing homes in Great Britian,[9] facilities that differ markedly from those in the

United States and are not typical in Britain, either. One way of describing this difference is by reference to the overworked "medical model" as compared with a "social model" for setting policies and organizing practices and social life in the institution. Whereas the typical pattern of nursing home organization is largely similar to that of a hospital, or more generally, a medical facility, these British nursing homes are organized more as a social facility. As in the typical nursing home, the residents are ill, ailing, infirm, mentally impaired, or incontinent, yet are able to perform a variety of tasks for themselves, including, for some, meal preparation. The residents are not only allowed but encouraged to make virtually every decision that affects their daily life and activity, except, of course, those requiring medical expertise. Thus they have liberty to choose the furniture in their rooms, to decide for themselves when to wake up in the morning and when to retire at night (even if they wish to stay up as late as 2 A.M.), and to make various other choices and decisions in their everyday lives. These British nursing homes thus strive to maximize the privacy, the autonomy, and the decisionmaking of their residents in an effort to create an atmosphere as similar as possible to that which the elderly persons enjoyed prior to entering. One especially striking feature is that residents are allowed to fight and squabble with one another, which enables them to vent their frustrations and emotions in ways they have experienced all their lives.

This social model has its value trade-offs, of course: what is a gain for the residents in their freedom, autonomy, and privacy amounts to a loss for staff in being able to run things as smoothly and efficiently as possible. The more choices and decisions that are left to the residents, the harder it is for staff to plan and organize the daily routine, since individual residents' wants and needs may vary substantially. It is apparently also true that the bias against paternalism is frequently difficult for the staff to accept, accustomed as they are to the norm in extended care facilities and hospitals, where the staff gives orders and constructs a regimen, and patients are expected to comply. One very positive benefit for residents of these facilities is improvement in depression, one of the most troubling and intractable characteristics of elderly persons.

If careful, empirical observation reveals that changes of this sort in the social structure of a facility for the elderly do indeed yield such benefits, then it is ethically desirable to make an effort to bring about such changes. Benefits to the residents clearly would seem to outweigh inconvenience and reduced efficiency of the staff, and although practical difficulties must always be heeded in any recommendations for change, this particular experience suggests another area for further research that might improve care and treatment of the elderly in extended care facilities.

NOTES TO CHAPTER 8

1. National Institute on Aging Task Force, "Senility Reconsidered: Treatment Possibilities for Mental Impairment in the Elderly," *Journal of the American Medical Association* 244 (1980): 259.
2. G.B. Kolata, "Clues to the Cause of Senile Dementia," *Science* 211 (1981): 1032.
3. National Institute on Aging Task Force, "Senility Reconsidered," pp. 259–263.
4. *Ibid.*, p. 260.
5. *Ibid.*
6. L.H. Roth, et al. "Tests of Competency to Consent to Treatment," *American Journal of Psychiatry* 134 (1977): 279–284.
7. *Ibid.*, pp. 283–284.
8. W.T.Reich, "Ethical Issues Related to Research Involving Elderly Subjects," *Gerontologist* 18 (1978): 333.
9. Presentation by Dr. Marvin Rosenberg delivered at The Hastings Center, Institute of Society, Ethics and the Life Sciences, Project on Health Policy and Geriatrics, May 13, 1981.

9 NURSES AND MORAL DISTRESS IN THE HOSPITAL

Andrew Jameton

Hospitals present a chiaroscuro pattern of beneficial and harmful practices. From one point of view, to labor in the hospital is to labor in the pits. Like Eugene O'Neill's Hairy Ape (the coal stoker at the ship's furnaces below deck), nurses, respiratory therapists, and residents stoke the furnaces of suffering under an unceasing fluorescent glare, along clattering halls coated not in soot, but painted pale green, white, or pink. Attending physicians, like wealthy passengers on the catwalk above, stop briefly to marvel at the spectacle and depart to the dining room. From another point of view, this picture is outrageously distorted. Health care is noble and beautiful. The health care team heals the sick and succors the dying. Intimate contact with human suffering elevates us. Medical techniques, although still not perfected, are glowing marvels compared to the dark remedies of the past. Health professionals express the most powerful tradition of humane ideals of any occupation.

Since urgent good and gruesome evil cohabit in the hospitals, nurses work in ambiguity and contradiction. Since they do both good and bad things to patients, nurses ask themselves whether the enterprise as a whole justifies their continuing cooperation with things that are, in their judgment, reprehensible. That someone else generally makes the decision to undertake a risky procedure does not relieve the feeling of complicity in wrong, since nurses are "hands on" in many procedures.

131

Nurses feel guilt and real moral distress when they perform procedures that they feel are morally wrong and can find no way to avoid them. Common instances causing this distress in nursing experiences are:

1. A nurse is assigned to perform a painful test on a child when the child is dying, and it seems to the nurse that the test is irrelevant to the child's welfare.
2. A nurse in the adult intensive care unit is assigned to care for a patient whom the nurse believes is dead. A machine pumps the chest and the heart beats, but the brain is dead.
3. In the newborn intensive care unit, a nurse cares for a severely damaged infant that she feels in her heart cannot survive. She punctures its heel each day to take blood tests.
4. The nurse is tending a patient who is about to have surgery and who has signed the consent forms for it. Yet the nurse suspects from the patient's conversation that the patient has no comprehension of the seriousness of the choice.
5. A surgeon fails to wash his hands before examining a patient in the Intensive Care Unit (ICU), and ignores the nurse's reminder.[1]

These cases are more than failures to realize an ideal: They involve what nurses judge to be morally wrong. Thus, nurses can be very critical of the hospitals in which they work: "I wonder if we should even work here. It seems like an immoral place to work," said one Coronary Care Unit nurse just before she quit her job. Another nurse made similar remarks: "Politics, or catering to the doctors—that's what counts around here."

There is an overriding feeling of doing McDonald's nursing.[2] But nurses work at hospitals and contribute to the setting. Are staff nurses to blame for what is going on? Is this painful sense of guilt that nurses feel legitimate? The American Nurses' Association (ANA) "Code for Nurses" gives a straightforward partial answer to this question. The code states unequivocally: "The nurse acts to safeguard the client and the public when health care and safety are affected by incompetent, unethical, or illegal practice of any person."[3] It is unprofessional, therefore, to cooperate in acts that, in the nurse's judgment, unethically impose risks on patients. But this is merely the beginning of the inquiry. Does failure to meet this duty require one to feel guilty? What can one do when ethical dilemmas arise? Do nurses really have any choice about these things? To examine these questions, consider a common but difficult case: What can and should nurses do about incompetent medical practitioners?

DEALING WITH MEDICAL INCOMPETENCE

There is an old joke that beds are dangerous because so many people die in them. From that point of view, hospital beds are particularly dangerous. In 1964, a study showed that 20 percent of patients on the wards of a teaching hospital suffered iatrogenic harm.[4] Iatrogenic illness is that caused by unsound medical (or nursing) interventions. In a more recent study reported in 1981, the combined medical, nursing, and other health care error rate was 36 percent. Nine percent of these errors were life-threatening, and 2 percent of these killed patients (or 0.7 percent of all patients admitted). This is a *conservative* estimate; if there was any doubt about the medical source of an untoward event, it was not counted. The authors attributed the 150 percent increase in errors since 1964 to increasingly complex medical technology.[5] A recent study of surgical errors with adverse outcomes found fewer errors but worse consequences. It found a 1 percent error rate, an overall mortality rate of 55 percent, average excess hospitals costs of $40,000 per client, and an average of 40 days excess hospitalization.[6]

These studies do not show that patients should stay out of the hospital; they may have been in worse condition if they had stayed at home, but the studies show that coping with errors is part of everyday hospital work. What should nurses do when they detect mistakes in their own work and in that of other nurses, physicians, or other hospital workers? To consider the issue, let us look at an extreme case: not simply the excusable mistakes of a competent clinician, but the chronic mistakes of an incompetent one. The following incident took place in the late 1970s in a medium-sized private teaching hospital:

> Dr. Hyde performed four surgeries at Mt. Citadel Hospital during a four-month period. All four were for slowly growing cancers in debilitated elderly patients. All four patients died slow, painful deaths in the Intensive Care Unit. There was a consensus among the ICU nurses and residents that Dr. Hyde performed the surgeries for marginal indications, that he performed them badly, and that he atrociously mismanaged their follow-up care in the unit. Said Nurse Robin, "He wrote orders that were just ridiculous."

How did the ICU staff nurses deal with this problem?

The ICU nurses did their best to see that each of Dr. Hyde's patients got the best care possible under the circumstances. They carried out the instructions of residents as quickly as possible and delayed filling Dr. Hyde's less competent changes in their orders.

They did not complain through hospital channels. In their opinion, the head nurse and the medical director were weak and would not help. The residents concurred in this judgment and so complained through very indirect channels. Staff were not yet sure whose side the new Director of Nursing was on. Moreover, seeing her would require going over the head nurse's head.

They hesitated to use any "outside" channels, not because they feared losing their jobs, but they did fear a possible libel suit. When they looked at the case records, they could not find any obvious defects in them. Only the patients were in bad shape.

They did not discuss their concerns with Dr. Hyde because they hated him. Everybody hated him. Besides they were sure that he knew he was incompetent, and his air of theatrical insincerity discouraged frank discussion.

They did not discuss it with any of the families. Only Mr. Apple had family actively involved in his care. His sister suspected that Dr. Hyde was not managing the case well. The nurses stood by when she asked Dr. Hyde how Mr. Apple was doing. "He's doing fine," said Dr. Hyde.

The sister asked Ms. Robin privately later, "Why is he still in a coma?" "What could I say?" commented Ms. Robin months later, "The patient has rotted for a month. It is too late to say, 'Somebody blew it.' I am just a nurse. All I know is that his patients don't do well. At this point, confidence in the doctor was about all the health care we had to offer."

The nursing staff hoped that Mr. Apple's sister would ask if a second opinion was needed. When they induced her to ask this, the nurses said, "YES!" The sister consulted the Director of Surgery at the hospital, an excellent surgeon whom the nurses regarded as beyond reproach. But he whitewashed the case in his report to the sister and in his notes in the record. No problems were mentioned about the indications for surgery, the surgery itself, or the post surgical management. Nurse Robin said, "I felt physically ill."

The staff nurses engaged in a number of rituals to ease their tension. When Dr. Hyde's four patients filled half the ICU beds and Mr. Apple's sister came to visit, the staff lined up all four patients in exactly the same position with their respirator hoses in exactly parallel alignment. They labelled that part of the ICU "The Dr. Hyde Memorial Isolation Room." When the last patient died, Ms. Robin cowled herself in a sheet like a nun "to escort Mr. Apple to his Heavenly Rest."

Before Dr. Hyde got to a fifth patient, a quiet, informal agreement was reached between him and the Chief of Surgery: he was not to perform any surgeries at Mt. Citadel without first consulting closely with the Chief, and all surgery had to be performed with another surgeon.

A month after Mr. Apple died, Ms. Robin ran into his sister on the street. She asked again what the nurses thought of Dr. Hyde. Ms. Robin still could not bring herself to say anything critical. That she never talked openly with his sister remains for her one of the most painful and doubtful issues about her own actions. Ms. Robin asks, "What do you do when you know what you have no right to know?"[7]

Cases like these are extremely painful and complex. There are three things that we should ask about this particular case. First, what was Ms. Robin's obligation to say something to the patient or to do something about the problem? Second, what courses of actions were available to her? And third, did she really have a choice?

There are many things she considered and should have considered in ascertaining her obligation:

Was she sure the doctor was incompetent? Absolute certainty that there is a problem is not required. In health care, one always has to work under conditions of uncertainty. The unit may have been in the grip of coincidence and mass hysteria. But since Dr. Hyde's orders appeared "ridiculous" to everyone, surely there was adequate evidence to raise the issue.

Of course, one has to be cautious in making such judgments. In another case, a nursing student tried to get a resident to order a lower dose of a hazardous antibiotic. As it turned out, dangerous side effects occurred. The client became deaf and suffered kidney failure. The nurse had already protested to the chief of medicine before the antibiotic was administered. Hindsight proved her right no more than the patient's recovery would have vindicated the resident.

Was this an issue of protecting the patient? The ANA Code is clear that protection is owed to the patient, but in this case the primary harm had already been done. It was too late to interfere with the surgery. Yet, during his stay in the ICU, further harm to Mr. Apple might have been prevented by discussing the issue with his sister. After he was dead, or nearly dead, protection was no longer the issue; instead, the issue became one of protection for future patients.

The duty to protect patients could call for some strange actions. For example, if Ms. Robin saw that a *fifth* patient were scheduled for the same kind of surgery with Dr. Hyde, would she have a duty to speak to that patient?

Would the patient or the family lose faith in health care? We do not know what would have happened. Perhaps the sister would have lost faith in the nurse for challenging her confidence in the doctor, but in this case confidence already seemed weak. Moreover, is health care something that should be an article of faith? Good results are sometimes obtained by admitting errors to patients. Such admissions help clients better understand what is happening to them when unexpected side effects occur. Or patients may appreciate the trust shown them through frankness.

Does the patient want to know? If the patient asks a question, then there is good reason to think that the patient wants to know the answer. Mr. Apple's sister asked. If the patient does not ask, matters are less clear. Some hold that the patient's views should prevail, and so we should not challenge patients who choose incompetent clinicians. They know more about their needs than we do as observers, and they may be getting things from their clinicians that we do not recognize.

This position will not do, however. It is part of the practice of a profession to make judgments about other practitioners of it. Dr. Hyde may have had charm, but his incompetence as a surgeon was also relevant to the patient. Assessing basic competencies of practitioners is not like trying to judge acupuncturists or faith healers, who claim a different *kind* of competence. Ms. Robin is a nurse; Dr. Hyde is a physician. They are not members of the same profession. But their professions overlap, so she was in a position to make judgments about his competence.

Would disclosure expose Ms. Robin to personal risks? Every health professional who things of whistle-blowing rightly worries about retaliation. She could become seen as a troublemaker and lose the confidence and cooperation of other nurses and physicians. Moreover, patients are natural hostages for retaliation. A physician may react to a request for a second opinion by dropping the patient or creating difficulties with a subsequent patient. Nurses who blow the whistle are sometimes fired—never for blowing the whistle, but for some unrelated infraction of the rules. Would this have happened in the above case? Ms. Robin's view of Dr. Hyde was widely shared, but apparently the impulse to speak to Mr. Apple's sister was not, since no one else spoke to her. We simply do not know what would have happened.

Are there any conflicting obligations? Hospital workers owe loyalty to other workers, but in this case, Ms. Robin *hated* Dr. Hyde. If she owed him any loyalty, it was of the most abstract kind, based merely on his occupation. She had a much stronger relationship with Mr. Apple's sister, and perhaps even with the comatose Mr. Apple. Discussing the matter with the client would also help to break down the professional/patient barrier, an ever present obstacle to nurse/patient relations.

Were her motives pure? It would not do for health professionals to go about blaming each other for the problems of health care. Was she displacing on Dr. Hyde her justified hostility to physicians as a group and her own guilt over the inadequacies of Mt. Citadel Intensive Care? Or did she decide not to disclose because she wanted to avoid trouble for herself and protect herself? These are the things one learns about only through time and by looking at one's other choices: Does one admit one's *own* errors? Is one complaining about everything?

In summary, there is a strong case here for disclosure:

Mr. Apple's sister asked for information; Ms. Robin had information of which she was fairly confident; protection of the patient was the issue. Countervailing considerations and possibilities were present, but they were not as strong in this case as in many others.[8] In spite of their distress, something Ms. Robin and other nurses did worked. They brought the case, admittedly indirectly, to the attention of the Chief of Surgery. Although he was unwilling to act for the record, he restricted Dr. Hyde's activities.

COOPERATION IN WRONGDOING

Hospital staff nurses rarely undertake on their own initiative or as team leaders what they regard as questionable procedures. They usually find themselves involved in bad practice through cooperation with others. The case above was just one extreme example. General principles to keep in mind in setting limits on cooperation are these:

1. *What is the seriousness of the harm involved?* The more serious the danger posed to this patient or to future patients, the stronger the call to action. The practitioner causing the harm may be

competent, incompetent, well-meaning, or uncaring—these considerations are not as relevant as the amount of harm.

2. *Does this happen often?* The more chronic the problem in one's institution, the more reason one has to address it.

3. *Are there ways to prevent the harm or future occurrences?* Refusing to participate or speaking to the head nurse or supervisor may prevent the incident or lead to changes in the future. Even if there is no recourse, some acts are so wrong that one should not cooperate in them, whatever the consequences.

4. *What is the nurse's role in causing the harm?* One's responsibility grows as one becomes more closely involved in causing the harm. A nurse is responsible for administering a harmful medication, although the act is done at the instruction of a physician. Although this is a fine point, the nurse who cares for a patient after a questionable surgery is in a morally safer position than a nurse who prepares the patient for surgery.[9]

5. *What is the nurse's attitude with regard to the harm?* A nurse who wholeheartedly supports a questionable procedure is more actively responsible for it than a nurse who acts reluctantly.[10]

In brief, nurses are in general *accountable* for harmful practices in which they are involved, even though they do not initiate them. As the profession becomes more autonomous, the responsibility of nurses for health practices increases. Thus, if health care continues to have problems, nurses will become responsible for them not merely as accomplices, but as principle agents.

HOW TO PROCEED WITH COMPLAINTS

What should one do about one's own mistakes or those of others? What should one do first? The ANA "Code for Nurses" is specific about what steps to take.

First, "concern should be expressed to the person carrying out the questionable practice and attention called to the possible detrimental effects upon the client's welfare." The next step, if needed, is "the responsible administrative person." Then, "if indicated, the practice should then be reported to the appropriate authority within the institution, agency, or larger system." The Code states that such an authority or mechanism for reporting to an authority should have "an established mechanism for the reporting and handling of incompetent, unethical, or illegal practice within the employment setting so that such reporting can go through official channels and be done without fear of reprisal." The Code says that "local units of the professional association should be prepared to provide assistance." Finally, if problems persist, "the problem should be reported to other appropriate authorities such as the practice committees of the appropriate professional organizations or the legally constituted bodies concerned with licensing of specific categories of health workers or professional practitioners."[11]

One of the problems is that there are so *many* ways one can proceed. And there are more ways than the ANA mentions: One can speak to the client or the client's family. One can go to the courts or newspapers. Or one could go to one's union.

Virtually all hospitals have established a mechanism of filing *incident reports.* Nurses are expected to file these reports on every untoward incident—a bad drug reaction, a fall or spill, a drunken practitioner. Hospitals like to have these for a documentary basis if any legal actions occur and for discussing changes in procedures. They have defects, however: Most incident reports are simply filed. They are not an instrument useful for nurses in discussing their mistakes.[12] Instead, they are an instrument of administration. And filing an incident report on another practitioner can invite retaliation.

Coping with bad *medical* practice can be an extremely delicate matter. Not only are nurses relatively powerless in relationship to physicians in these matters, but physicians regard the problem of bad medical practice as one of extreme delicacy. Most procedures are complex and mined with legal pitfalls.[13]

In California, for example, the Board of Medical Quality Assurance oversees licensure and discipline of physicians. It has a procedure by which *anyone* can make a complaint simply by filing a form. The Board will always respond with an investigation. The Civil Code

provides nearly absolute immunity for persons who communicate ' . . . information . . . to any hospital, hospital medical staff, professional society, medical or dental school, professional licensing board or division, committee or panel of such licensing board, peer review committee, or underwriting committee . . . when such communication is intended to aid in the evaluation of the qualifications, fitness, character, or insurability of a practitioner of the healing arts and does not represent as true any matter not reasonably believed to be true.'[14]

In spite of these many options, and in spite of written assurances of protection, most people view whistle-blowing as a hazardous and ineffective venture:

> 'I don't know why I bother to fill this out,' she complained. 'I've worked in this unit for more than seven years, and in that time I've filed exactly three reports about medical practice. Nothing is ever done . . . You document what you observed, and you darn well better have proof. You know it doesn't matter when a doctor is complaining about a nurse. No one asks for proof of what he says, but if I complain about a physician's practice, I'm just not taken seriously. . . . Nothing is ever done.'[15]

Are nurses right in this judgment? In spite of these problems, 80 percent of respondents to an *R.N.* survey reported that they have been able to take effective action in response to medical errors.[16] Or, if procedures were used more widely and actively, would the air clear and action be taken? The only way to find out is to use these mechanisms and to create new ones.

CONSCIENTIOUS OBJECTION

All of the above forms of recourse are *verbal*. Another recourse is simply to refuse to cooperate with a procedure even if ordered to do it. The legal model for refusal is called *conscientious objection*. Refusals to cooperate in employment situations are similar where one's noncooperation violates the employer's policies or the conditions of one's employment, and where one's protest is based on issues of conscience.

Civil disobedience in order to make a public point about a moral issue has been prominent in the birth control movement. Emma Goldman, Van Kleek Allison, Margaret Sanger, and Ethel Byrne all violated laws in the early part of the century to marshal support for the legalization of contraception. While she was in jail, Margaret Sanger tried to distribute birth control information among other prisoners.[17]

The issue of conscientious objection has arisen recently in connection with abortion. Although abortions are legal, some nurses strongly object to them on grounds of conscience. Nurses who object should not be required to cooperate with them, not because they might provide bad care, but because they should not be required to cooperate in what they regard as evil. Thelma Schorr, for example, argues:

> There are many nurses who see an abortion as an unconscionable act, and certainly they should never be placed in the position of having to nurse patients who have chosen to have their pregnancies terminated. Just as a patient's freedom to choose must be respected, so must a nurse's. But it is also that nurse's responsibility to protect both the patient's freedom and her own by refusing to work in a situation which she finds morally offensive.[18]

Institutions should make arrangements to make conscientious non-cooperation possible. For example, the International Labour Conference recommends:

> 18. Nursing personnel should be able to claim exemption from performing specific duties, without being penalized, where performances would conflict with their religious, moral, or ethical convictions and where they inform their supervisor in good time of their objection so as to allow the necessary alternative arrangements to be made to ensure that essential nursing care of patients is not affected.[19]

Analogously, bad nursing and medical practice also can be seen as issues of conscience: if not of private conscience, at least of professional conscience. It is not at all unusual for nurses to refuse to carry out questionable orders by physicians. Physicians often carry out the orders themselves without much conflict. The nurse may say, "I won't give an injection for this much morphine; you'll have to do it yourself." The physician says, "All right. I'll do it."

If one felt strongly about an issue, one could go further. A nurse could say, "Anyone who comes near this patient will do so at their peril," and physically prevent procedures from being done. In 1974, the Feminist Women's Health Center in Los Angeles stole the equipment from a substandard abortion clinic in order to prevent its operation.[20] In another case, nursing aides at a nursing home sued their employers because supervisors were ordering aides to engage in abusive procedures, such as disciplining patients with cold showers.

Nurses and physicians have found highly varied ways in which to cope with conflicts between their standards of practice and the rules under which their work is conducted. For example, it is still the law in California that babies' eyes must be washed with silver nitrate as a prophylactic against gonorrhea. In the judgment of many clinicians, this is unnecessary in many cases. When parents refuse to consent to the procedure, newborn units vary in their reactions: One unit insists on performing the procedure because it is required by law. If they have to, they sign and file the consent themselves. In another unit, they simply forget about it. In another, they carry out the procedure and do not tell the parents. In another, they document doing the procedure but do not do it. In another, they make up a very light wash of silver nitrate and wash it out very quickly. This variety of reactions indicates the depth and difficulty of finding ways to proceed when one is morally distressed and facing institutional constraints. Moral *distress* engenders moral *dilemmas*.

IS THERE REALLY A CHOICE?

Many of the institutional practices that we regret appear to us as contraints—like natural laws that limit our actions. There are many things we simply cannot do—for example, make a hospital committee listen when it won't. In some conceivable sense of *can*, perhaps, one can make it listen, but to do so would require nearly impossible quantities of energy and involve great personal risks or violations of principles one holds dear. Indeed, there are really two very different kinds of limits on our ability to choose: There are limits of physical and psychological possibility, and limits of conventions and ethics.

An important viewpoint on human possibility is articulated by Jean Paul Sartre, who wrote extensively about human freedom and responsibility.[21] He believed that we are completely free to choose, no matter what circumstances we are in. He emphasized that what ethics says one can and cannot do does not exhaust the possibilities open to one. Ethics, for example, says that we should not force a committee to listen to us by waving a gun at its members, but we still *can*.

He believed that most of us find this freedom awesome and frightening. It makes us responsible for everything that goes on around us. So we try to escape this freedom. We pretend to ourselves that we are forced to do things when we are not. When the nurse, for example, tells a patient "You must do this because the doctor ordered it," both the nurse and patient pretend that they must act because of the doctor's order, but in fact either one could make another choice.

We use ethics to escape from freedom. Sometimes a nurse will ask an ethicist "What should I do?" and the nurse is told that ethics does not give a definite answer. Instead of rejoicing that ethics leaves room for choice, the nurse regrets that there is no rule or principle that forces a choice. Sartre believed that there is no significant morality except that of honest choice and personal responsibility.

This is one of the deeper meanings of *accountability*. Nurses who work in the hospital are accountable for their choices there because they choose to work there when they could choose otherwise. Many nurses leave nursing precisely because they reject hospital working conditions. Burn out is partially a moral statement.

Sartre is not suggesting that everyone should leave nursing. The good that hospitals do must also be credited to one's account. It is a legitimate choice to stay in the hospital, to accomplish as much as one can there, and to struggle for changes. What Sartre wants to emphasize is that this is a *choice*, not a necessity.

Another point of view emphasizes the limits set by ethical claims of institutions. Immanuel Kant, for example, gives expression to this position: "Many affairs which are conducted in the interest of the community require a certain mechanism through which some members of the community must passively conduct themselves with artificial unanimity, so that the government may direct them to public ends, or at least prevent them from destroying those ends."[22]

The government is not the only institution that demands "artificial unanimity." Any large business enterprise requires the smooth cooperation of many persons to accomplish its ends, and hospitals are no exception. If the hospital were to become the site of daily discussions of the aims, goals, and morality of health care, there would be little time left for work. It is thus a difficult conflict for us to reconcile our conception of ourselves as autonomous agents with the need of major productive endeavors for orderly cooperation.

A very basic choice is forced on those who work in hospitals by the existence of prevalent and systematic problems in health care. If one fails to resist exploitation, incompetence, and corrupt practices, one becomes responsible for them. If one resists them, one enters conflict with conventional conceptions of behavior for employees and risks reprisals. One has to choose between complicity and self-sacrifice, or enter the uncomfortable middle ground of irony. Ethics does not give a clear answer as to which one must choose. Instead, one is free to move in the direction of the kind of world one personally desires to create.

RISKS AND PERSONAL SACRIFICES

Should nurses take risks or sacrifice personal interests for the sake of patient care? In any society, some sacrifice of one's interests is demanded of all. Paying taxes, engaging in politics, avoiding harm to others, and the like involve some sacrifice, but they are necessary contributions to the common good. If we did not generally make such contributions, we would all be worse off. Sacrifices thought of as *charity* or volunteer work are not usually required, but are generally praised. Such activities create personal rewards, but partly through personal costs.

Health care is a traditionally charitable enterprise, and it is traditionally honorable and ethical to make sacrifices for the health of patients. Exposing oneself to disease in order to care for the sick is a traditional health care virtue. Similarly, it is a virtue to risk one's job in order to protect one's patient.

Health *professionals* generally place the good of the patient first. That means that if my interests on occasion have to be sacrificed for the sake of the patient, then I should sacrifice them. How much one should sacrifice is unclear. One can extend oneself to levels of *sainthood* and *heroism.* Being extremes, such actions are necessarily rare. If heroism and sainthood were required, they would then be conventional and no longer exceptional.[23] They must then be morally *optional*. At the same time, our moral ideals stand ready to praise sainthood and acts of heroism and to make them meaningful.

Nurses in particular should be wary of the temptations of self-sacrifice. Nurses have traditionally been called upon to sacrifice themselves. Under calls to idealism, they have been asked to work long hours for low wages and to show deference to physicians—to bring them chairs and charts, not to benefit the patient, but to benefit the physicians. Self-abnegation by women nurses also confirms traditional sex discrimination. Self-sacrifice by nurses is thus best directed only toward patients and acts that strengthen nurses as a group. It is perhaps better to think in terms of acts of heroism rather than saintliness.[24]

The following considerations are useful in considering whether to take personal risks to avoid complicity in harming patients:

1. Personal sacrifice is justified only where there is some possibility that something may be achieved by it. That "something" can be interpreted broadly, such as avoiding complicity in wrongdoing.

2. The greater the risk of harm to the patient or to future patients, the greater the obligation to make some sacrifice (if needed and efficacious) to reduce the risk.

3. It is more important to think in terms of having a good defense for what one does than it is to think in terms of avoiding risks. It is hard to fault someone who: (a) acts sincerely, (b) gives clearly articulated reasons that others can understand, (c) consults with others in making a decision, and (d) acts publicly and on the record.

4. One should assess personal risk realistically. One should not frighten oneself into paralysis by tales of unlikely and horrendous consequences.

5. It is both prudent and morally acceptable to take steps to protect oneself. (It is helpful, for example, in a tightly managed hospital, not to be vulnerable on other grounds.)

6. What are others doing? If someone thinks something is morally wrong, there must be others who agree. Act collectively wherever possible.

7. Nursing is a profession, not a calling. It does not call for unlimited commitment.

8. Exposure of oneself to risks in order to protect patients is a well-established conventional obligation of the health professions.

ETHICS AND THE FUTURE OF NURSING PRACTICE

Bioethics came of age in a period of conflict and crisis in health care. Basic problems in the organization of health care created among practitioners many questions about the ethics of their work. Moral uncertainties, distress, and dilemmas testified to the depth of reactions of nurses and other health professionals to this crisis.

These moral problems call for two very different but closely related responses. On one hand, they call for better philosophical and intellectual analysis. They call for clearer consciousness of what the problems are, clearer statements of conflicting principles, and thorough efforts to analyze them reflectively. On this work, philosophers can be most helpful.

On the other hand, this approach is limited. Distinctions can only become so subtle before they become laughable. A choice in a dilemma may be painful, but as well-resolved for the moment by a toss of a coin as by nicely stated arguments. Instead, we need to inquire why we are caught in these dilemmas at all. Why is there a conflict between loyalty to professionals and to patients? Why do life-saving methods reduce the quality of life? Why can we do so little about prevention? Where does the doctor/nurse game come from? We need to be conscious of the conditions that create ethical dilemmas and struggle to change them. The solution to moral problems is not merely finding a new intellectual statement; it is creating new modes of life and work. In this, philosophers must follow the lead of nurses and the nursing profession.

Articulation of moral principles and solutions to moral problems thus require some care. If we use our ideas about ethics to set hard-edged and unrealistic ideals, or if we use them to articulate principles meaninglessly distant from life, we only set ourselves up for disillusionment. Such exercises may be valuable as exhortation or analysis, but they do not express what we think we *really* should do. On the other hand, if we were so realistic in our ethical thinking as to endorse the world as it is, we would fail again at ethical thinking: We know that the world is not as it should be.

The world will change. Nursing practice and our organizations for providing health care will change. Present dilemmas will pass and others come to the fore. It is hard to guess what is possible in the future. For example, nurses are gaining in power and influence, and conceptions of nursing as a profession have been increasingly accepted. But this is taking place just at a time when professions in health care are under attack from many directions. It is hard to say what will result from this struggle.

What we choose to say in our moral principles and solutions to problems is important to the struggle by nurses for power and recognition. Ethics should support our choices for the future and should express what is possible. It should strengthen nurses, rather than limit and discourage them. At the same time, by supporting one direction more than another, it can make that direction possible by leading us toward it and focusing our energies in that direction. Ethics should express what we hope for in what we sense is possible.

Nursing has been an important humanizing force in health care. Compassion for the ill and dying, protection for the vulnerable, health education, and skillful treatment of the sick are all basic human goods that express our idealism about the ability of human beings to care for each other. There are many forces that threaten our ability to express humane ideals in the world—economic inequality, limited resources, burgeoning military weaponry, sexism, racism, and so on. By carrying a tradition of humane ideals, nurses can be friends to both humanity and themselves. Ethics supports the power of nursing in its expression of this tradition.

NOTES TO CHAPTER 9

1. For recent rates of hand-washing, see Richard K. Albert and Francis Condie, "Hand-Washing Patterns in Medical Intensive-Care Units," *The New England Journal of Medicine*, 304 (1981): 1465-1466. In relationship to patient contacts, nurses wash their hands about twice as often as physicians. But since nurses have the bulk of contact with patients, most unwashed contacts are with nurses. Respiratory therapists are *tops* at hand-washing.
2. Frances J. Storlie, "Burnout: The Elaboration of a Concept," *American Journal of Nursing* 79 (1979): 2108.
3. The AMA code has a similar provision: "A physician should deal honestly with patients and colleagues, and strive to expose those physicians deficient in character or competence, or who engage in fraud or deception (AMA, 1980)."
4. Elihu M. Schimmel, "The Hazards of Hospitalization," *Annals of Internal Medicine* 60 (1964): 100-110.
5. Knight Steel, et al., "Iatrogenic Illness on a General Medical Service at a University Hospital," *The New England Journal of Medicine* 304 (1981): 638-642.
6. Nathan P. Couch, et al., "The High Cost of Low-Frequency Events: The Anatomy and Economics of Surgical Mishaps," *The New England Journal of Medicine* 304 (1981): 634-637.
7. I chose a nurse/doctor problem because such problems are so often discussed by nurses. I am unsure whether the incompetence of other nurses is mentioned less often because it is a simpler or a more difficult problem.
8. This judgment is itself a form of "second-guessing," arrived at over several years' contemplation. I was present during the last weeks of this case. Should I have done more about it? If so, what? Dr. Hyde is still in practice. Should I do something now?
9. In this and the next point, I am reflecting a distinction made in some Catholic ethics texts between *formal* and *material* cooperation. To cooperate in evil *formally* is either to choose or to desire the evil act itself, or to cooperate knowingly in actions that are a means to that evil act. To cooperate *materially* is to be involved not as a means and not to wish for

the evil outcome. I *formally* cooperate when I loan my brother my car when he asks me if he can use it to rob a bank. If he comes to me after the robbery and asks me to hide him, and this is the first I have heard of the robbery, hiding him would only be *material* cooperation. Formal cooperation is morally more culpable than material cooperation. See Joseph B. McAllister, *Ethics: With Special Application to the Medical and Nursing Professions*, 2nd ed. (Philadelphia: W.B. Saunders Company, 1955), pp. 97–98.

10. One cannot find permanent refuge in mental reservations (except under the most repressive conditions). Chronic reluctance eventually becomes bad faith and as morally problematic as wholehearted cooperation in evil.

11. American Nurses' Association, "Code for Nurses with Interpretative Statement" (Kansas City: 1976).

12. Physicians practice the regular ritual of the Morbidity and Mortality conference. In this conference, physicians confess their errors and discuss them openly and critically. This is a way of improving practice and displaying frankness, humility, and competence. See Charles L. Bosk, "Occupational Rituals in Patient Management," *The New England Journal of Medicine* 303 (1980): 71–76. To the best of my knowledge, nurses have no similar protected, regular setting in which to openly discuss mistakes.

13. William E. Mitchell, Jr., "How to Deal with Poor Medical Care," *Journal of the American Medical Association* 236 (1976): 2875–2877, describes some sound procedures and considerations for dealing with poor medical care. The procedures also reflect the difficulty in getting anything done.

14. California Medical Association and Board of Medical Quality Assurance, *Physician Responsibility . . . A Joint Statement*, January 1980 Sacramento, California: 5. This pamphlet is quoting from California Civil Code, Section 43.8.

15. Storlie, "Burnout," p. 2110.

16. Linda Stanley, "Dangerous Doctors: What to Do When the M.D. is Wrong," *R.N.* 42, no. 3 (March 1979): 25.

17. Edward H. Madden and Peter H. Hare, "Civil Disobedience in Health Services," in Warren T. Reich, ed., *Encyclopedia of Bioethics* Vol. IV (New York: The Free Press, 1978), p. 159.

18. Thelma Schorr, "Issues of Conscience, *American Journal of Nursing* 72 (1972): 61.

19. International Labour Conference, "Text of the Recommendation Concerning Employment and Conditions of Work and Life of Nursing Personnel, Submitted by the Drafting Committee," *Provisional Record*, Sixty-Third Session (Geneva, 1977), p. 21B/5.

20. Madden and Hare, "Civil Disobedience," p. 160.

21. For a brief account of Sartre's views, see "Existentialism is a Humanism," in George Novack, ed., *Existentialism Versus Marxism: Conflicting Views on Humanism* (New York: Dell Publishing Co., 1966): 70–84.

22. Immanuel Kant, *Foundations of the Metaphysics of Morals and What is Enlightenment*, trans. Lewis White Beck (Indianapolis: The Bobbs–Merrill Company, Inc., 1959), p. 87.

23. J.O. Urmson, "Saints and Heroes," in Joel Feinberg, ed., *Moral Concepts* (New York: Oxford University Press, 1970), pp. 60-73.

24. Saintliness has stronger connotations of moral goodness than heroism. A hero or heroine can be noble but not necessarily moral. Heroism can be episodic, but saintliness requires a long track record. Physicians are more often described as heroic than saintly, and we have such concepts as *heroic intervention* and *heroic medicine*. Saintliness has been more closely associated with nursing, especially as a result of nursing's early associations with religious orders.

III COOPERATIVE METHODS FOR RESOLVING VALUE CONFLICTS IN HEALTH CARE

Bioethicists discuss the problems of medical ethics, but do not usually experience them directly. In contrast, these problems are the daily fare of physicians, nurses, physical therapists, and others who work in the health care system. It is therefore surprising that more inter-disciplinary work between bioethicists and health care providers has not been initiated by either party. The four chapters in this section address this anomaly in differing ways. The first and third chapters provide illustrations of such collaborative work, the author of the second lays the groundwork for interdisciplinary work in a specific area of value conflict, and the author of the fourth argues that such work is essential and overdue.

In "On the Definition and Criterion of Death" James L. Bernat, Charles M. Culver, and Bernard Gert, two physicians and a philoso-pher, confront the issue of the definition of death. Recent techno-logical advances have raised new and troubling controversies that focus on the nature of death. Can a patient whose cardiopulmonary and respiratory systems are being maintained by support systems be considered dead? Could an organ be removed from the body of such a patient for transplant? Is a person who has lost all higher brain function dead even if there is spontaneous breathing and heartbeat? These questions and a corresponding array of related ethical ques-tions are generated by unclarity about the nature and definition of death.

The authors begin by distinguishing the *definition* of death, which is nonmedical and part of our ordinary conceptual framework, from the *criterion* of death, which, though physiological in nature, must be understandable by laypeople. According to the authors, death is defined "as the permanent cessation of functioning of the organism as a whole." They next compare two competing criteria for this permanent cessation, viz., the loss of cardiopulmonary function versus the total and irreversible loss of whole brain function. Due to recent technological advances, they argue that the loss of cardiopulmonary function does not necessarily correlate with permanent nonfunctioning of the organism as a whole, and so the criterion of death should be the irreversible cessation of all brain function. Nonetheless, a sufficient *test* of when this criterion is satisfied will be "the irreversible cessation of spontaneous respiratory and circulatory functions . . . in the absence of any medical evidence to the contrary." By clarifying the *definition* of death, positing a single *criterion* for death, and exploring the relationship between this criterion and the usual medical *tests* of death, Bernat, Culver, and Gert have clarified an issue that is of concern to lawyers, physicians, bioethicists, and the public at large. At the same time, their work illustrates precisely the kind of careful interdisciplinary collaboration that we believe is needed to confront the troublesome ethical dilemmas that arise in the practice of medicine. Charles M. Culver and Bernard Gert have continued their interdisciplinary collaboration in *Philosophy in Medicine: Conceptual and Ethical Issues in Medicine and Psychiatry* (Oxford University Press, 1982).

Bart Gruzalski's essay, "When to Keep Patients Alive Against Their Wishes," is not a *result* of collaborative work, but rather argues for and concludes with a *call for* collaborative work in the treatment of burn victims. The ethical controversy here is what to do when a severe burn victim wants to be allowed to die but the staff believes the patient should be kept alive. Gruzalski begins by describing the "life-maintenance strategy" that prescribes keeping such patients alive until they can act independently on their own assessments of the value of their lives and, if they wish, commit suicide. He contrasts this strategy with a "case-by-case strategy" that rests on the claim that each such case is unique and is to be assessed on its own merits without reference to any policies that treat patients as if they are similar and require similar care. Gruzalski rejects the case-by-case strategy because it leaves these life and death decisions ungrounded in anything except the intuitions of house staff that may change from day to day and may differ from institution to institution. At exploring the contributions of both the Kantian and utilitarian ethical accounts to this issue, Gruzalski also rejects the life-maintenance strategy because, in part, it fails to distinguish between two different patient assessments of such paternalistic interventions: (1) that life is now worth living, and (2) that it was worth the pain and stress of treatment to stay alive. According to Gruzalski, a justifiable paternalistic intervention must satisfy several conditions, among them that the patient is likely to affirm that the treatment was worthwhile. On the basis of this conceptual point, which also corresponds to the Kantian and the utilitarian accounts of moral obligation, Gruzalski calls for a collaborative research into how those patients who have been kept alive against their wishes assess their treatment. Depending on the results of this collaborative research, we may uncover an objective basis for deciding in many cases when to treat burn victims against their wishes and when not to do so. To fail to proceed with such an investigation is to be unresponsive to the conceptual and ethical considerations that apply in these cases and, Gruzalski concludes, is, to be willing to take the chance of making life and death decisions on the basis of values and intuitions that may have little to do with the values and character of the patients involved.

In "Technology Assessment in Medical Care: Appraisal and Conflict Resolution" Seymour Perry shifts from a discussion of specific ethical problems to a more general discussion of how we as a society are to evaluate new technological developments in health care. Perry describes two institutional responses to this important need. The first is the National Institutes of Health's use of Consensus Development panels to assess new developments. The purpose of these panels, according to Perry, is to synthesize the best current opinions to assist medical professionals in clinical decisionmaking. These consensus panels bring together researchers, health care consumers, clinical specialists, and representatives of interested groups to assess specific technologies or health care policies. In so doing, interdisciplinary and pluralistic collaborative evaluations of health care developments result.

Perry's second illustration of collaborative assessments of such developments is the activities of the National Center for Health Care Technology. According to Perry, the Center acts primarily as a catalyst to bring together the various groups and individuals whose expertise and values would be relevant to a proper assessment. Once again, the result is the kind of interdisciplinary work that must be done to cope effectively with the value conflicts generated by the development of new health care technologies. In closing, Perry cites the criticisms of the National Center that were made by the AMA and the Health Industry Manufacturer's Association and that contributed to the demise of the agency. Perry argues that these criticisms were effectively answered by the record of the Center since its founding in 1978.

In the closing essay in this volume, "An Agenda For Medical Ethics," Samuel Gorovitz briefly reviews the history of medical ethics, describes the current taxonomy of issues being discussed, and identifies two reasons for the dissatisfaction some have with medical ethics. The first is that some people expect too much of medical ethics. But it is the second source of dissatisfaction that Gorovitz emphasizes, viz., that bioethicists and clinical practitioners come to the problems with such different objectives and backgrounds that what one finds gratifying, the other finds unsatisfactory. Gorovitz recommends that we

> close the gap between the clinician's approach to medical ethics and the philosopher's approach by embarking on a new agenda of inquiry into ethical problems in health care delivery, conducted as cooperative ventures by those who could responsibly be classified as 'bioethicists' working with appropriate colleagues in clinical practice. . . .

The research he suggests would not address problems of purely theoretical interest, but instead would address ongoing problems in health service delivery and health policy. Such work, according to Gorovitz, will also put some overdue attention on the problems that arise in the interaction between consumer and provider and also on the policy issues that shape the character of health services in the United States. Gorovitz provides three illustrations of how such collaborative research might be carried out and lists twenty-three areas of possible further work. Some of these areas—the issue of physician impairment, the issue of health care for the elderly, and the issue of honoring a patient's refusal of treatment—have been the subject of individual chapters in this volume. Another of these areas—the extent to which health care planners should attempt to deal with the nonmedical factors that are direct influences on the demand for and cost of health services—is the topic of our first section of chapters. Gorovitz convincingly states the case for an interdisciplinary approach to the problems of medical ethics, and it is just such a need that we have tried to begin to meet in assembling this volume.

10 ON THE DEFINITION AND CRITERION OF DEATH

James L. Bernat, Charles M. Culver,
and Bernard Gert

Much of the confusion arising from the current brain death controversy is due to the lack of rigorous separation and ordered formulation of three distinct elements: the definition of death, the medical criterion for determining that death has occurred, and the tests to prove that the criterion has been satisfied. This confusion can be reduced by the formulation of a definition of death that makes its ordinary meaning explicit, the choice of a criterion of death that shows that the definition has been fulfilled, and the selection of tests that indicate with perfect validity that the criterion is satisfied.

Another source of confusion has been introduced by the definitions of death that appear in legal dictionaries and the new statutory definitions of death. These do not account for what the layperson actually means by death, but merely state the criteria by which physicians legally determine when death has occurred. "Death," however, is not a technical term, but a common term in everyday use. We believe that a proper understanding of the ordinary meaning of the word or concept of death must be developed before a medical criterion of death is chosen. We must decide what is commonly meant by death before physicians can decide how to measure it.

Agreement on the correct definition and criterion of death is literally a life and death matter. Whether a spontaneously breathing pa-

Reprinted from *Annals of Internal Medicine* 94 no. 3 (March 1981).

tient in a chronic vegetative state is classified as dead or alive depends on our understanding of the definition of death. Even given the correct definition, the status of a patient with a totally and permanently dysfunctional brain who is being maintained on a ventilator depends on the criterion of death employed. Providing the definition is primarily a philosophical task; the choice of the criterion is primarily medical; and the selection of the tests to prove that the criterion is satisfied is solely a medical matter.

THE DEFINITION OF DEATH

Death as a Process or an Event

Death has often been described as a process rather than an event.[1] Evidence for this claim is found in the fact that a series of degenerative and destructive changes occurs in the tissues of an organism, usually following but sometimes prior to the irreversible cessation of spontaneous ventilation and circulation. These changes include: necrosis of brain cells, necrosis of other vital organ cells, cooling, rigor mortis, dependent lividity, and putrefaction. This process actually persists for years, even centuries, until the skeletal remains have disintegrated. Further, this process could be viewed as beginning with the failure of certain organ systems during life. Because these changes occur in a fairly regular and ineluctable fashion, stipulation of any particular point in this process as the moment of death seems arbitrary.

We believe that a definition of death stipulating that it occurs at a more or less definite time is preferable to a definition that makes death a process. If we regard death as a process, then either the process starts when the person is still living, which confuses the "process of death" with the process of dying, for we all regard someone who is dying as not yet dead, or the "process of death" starts when the person is no longer alive, which confuses death with the process of disintegration. Death should be viewed not as a process but as the event that separates the process of dying from the process of disintegration.

Although the definition of death as a process has value as a description of biological events and allows the avoidance of choosing between the various definitions of death discussed below, this view makes it impossible to precisely declare the time of death. This is not a trivial issue. There are pressing medical, legal, social, and religious reasons to declare the time of death with precision, including the interpretation of wills, burial times and procedures, mourning times, and decisions regarding the aggressiveness of medical support. There are no compensatory reasons to regard death as a process and not an event in the formulation of a definition of death. We shall say that the event of death occurs at some definite if not precisely determinable time.

Choices for a Definition of Death

The definition of death must encompass the common usage of the term, for "death" is a word used by everyone, and not primarily in the fields of medicine or law. Because certain facts are assumed in its common usage, we shall assume them as well and not attempt to answer the speculations of science fiction, such as if the brain continues to function independently of the rest of the organism.[2, 3] Thus, we assume that all and only living organisms can die, that the living can be distinguished from the dead with fairly good reliability, and that the moment when an organism leaves the former state and enters the latter can be determined. We know that literally death is permanent. Although there are religious theories about death involving the soul leaving the body, when a person dies, religious persons and secularists do not disagree in their ordinary use of the term "dead." We acknowledge that the body can remain physically intact for some time after death and some isolated parts of the organism may continue to function (for example, it is commonly believed that hair and nails continue to grow after death).

We define death as the permanent cessation of functioning of the organism as a whole. We do not mean the whole organism, for example, the sum of its tissue and organ parts, but rather the highly complex interaction of its organ subsystems. Also, the organism need not be whole or complete, it may have lost a limb or an organ (such as the spleen), but it still remains an organism. The spontaneous and innate interrelationship of all or most of the remaining subsystems and the interaction of the perhaps impaired organism with its environment is to be regarded as the functioning of the organism as a whole.

After the organism as a whole has permanently ceased to function, individual subsystems may function for a time. Although this is not true for spontaneous ventilation, which ceases either immediately after or just before the permanent cessation of functioning of the organism as a whole, it is true for spontaneous circulation, which with artificial ventilation may persist for up to two weeks after the organism as a whole has ceased to function.

The functioning of the organism as a whole means the spontaneous and innate activities carried out by the integration of all or most subsystems (for example, neuroendocrine control), and at least limited response to the environment (for example, temperature change and responses to light and sound). However, the integration of all of the subsystems is not necessary. Individual subsystems may be replaced (such as by pacemakers, ventilators, pressors) without changing the status of the organism as a whole.

Temperature regulation is one example of an activity of the organism as a whole. The control of this complex process is located in the hypothalamus and is important for normal maintenance of all cellular processes. It is lost when the organism as a whole has ceased to function. Although consciousness and cognition are sufficient evidence for the functioning of the organism as a whole in higher animals, even for them these functions are not necessary. Lower organisms never have consciousness and when a higher organism is comatose, proof of the functioning of the organism as a whole may still be evident, such as temperature regulation.

We believe that this definition encompasses the traditional meaning of death. Death is considered a biological occurrence not unique to humans, and other higher animals would be considered dead according to the same definition. As a biological phenomenon, death should apply equally to related species. When we talk of the death of a man we mean the same thing as we do when we talk of the death of a dog or a cat. This is supported by our ordinary use of the term death, by law, and by tradition. It is also in accord with social and religious practices and is not likely to be affected by future changes in technology. In their recent monograph, Grisez and Boyle[4] reach similar conclusions.

The definition of death as the irreversible loss of that which is essentially significant to the nature of man[5] seems initially very attractive, but we disagree with it on several grounds. First, it does not contain what is commonly meant by the term. According to common usage, stating that a person has lost that which is essentially significant to the nature of humans but is still alive is not self-contradictory. For example, we acknowledge that permanently comatose patients in chronic vegetative states are sufficiently brain-damaged that they have irreversibly lost all that is essentially significant to the nature of humans but we still consider them to be living (for example, Karen Ann Quinlan[6]).

The patients described by Brierley and associates[7] are also in this category. These patients had complete neocortical destruction with preservation of brainstem and diencephalic structures. They had isoelectric EEGs and were permanently comatose, although they had normal spontaneous breathing and brainstem reflexes; they were essentially in a permanent, severe, and chronic vegetative state.[8] They retained many of the vital functions of the organism as a whole, including neuroendocrine control and the control of circulation and breathing.

This proposed definition actually states what it is for an organism to cease to be a person rather than stating what it is for that organism which is a person to die. The concept "person" is not biological, but rather a concept defined in terms of certain kinds of abilities and qualities of awareness. It is inherently vague. Death is a biological concept. Thus in a literal sense, death can be applied directly only to biological organisms and not to persons. We do not object to the phrase "death of a person," but the phrase in common usage actually means the death of the organism which was the person. For example, one might overhear in the hospital wards, "The person in room 612 died last night." Obviously, in this common usage one is referring to the death of the organism that was a person. By our analysis, Veatch[9] and others have used the phrase "death of a person" metaphorically, applying it to an organism that has ceased to be a person but has not died.

Without question, consciousness and cognition are essential human attributes. If they are lost, life has lost its meaning. A patient in a chronic vegetative state is usually regarded as living only in the most basic, biological sense. But this basic biological sense is essential to our definition of death. We must not confuse the death of an organism which was a person, with an organism's ceasing to be a person. Immediately aware of the loss of personhood in these patients, we are repulsed by the idea of continuing to treat them as if they were persons. But considering these chronic vegetative patients as actually dead leads to some serious problems. First, a slippery slope condition would be introduced wherein the question could be asked: How much neocortical damage is necessary before we declare a patient dead? Surely patients in chronic vegetative states, although usually not totally satisfying the tests for neocortical destruction, have permanently lost their consciousness and cognition. Then what about the somewhat less severely brain damaged patient?

By considering permanent loss of consciousness and cognition as a criterion for ceasing to be a person and not for death of the organism as a whole, the slippery slope phenomenon is put where it belongs: not in the definition of death, but in the determination of possible grounds for nonvoluntary euthanasia. The justification of nonvoluntary euthanasia must be kept strictly separate from the definition of death. Most of us would like our organism to die when we cease to be persons, but this should not be accomplished by blurring the distinctions between biological death and the loss of personhood.

A practical problem also arises in considering chronically vegetative patients with spontaneous ventilation to be dead. Most would view burying such patients while they breathe and have a heartbeat as at least esthetically unacceptable. Then how will these vital signs be stopped and by whom? Disconnecting a ventilator from a recently declared dead patient fulfilling tests of permanent loss of whole brain functioning is one thing; suffocating a spontaneously breathing patient is another.

THE CRITERION OF DEATH

Having argued that the correct definition of death is permanent cessation of functioning of the organism as a whole, we will proceed to inspect the two competing criteria of death: the permanent loss of cardiopulmonary functioning and the total and irreversible loss of funtioning of the whole brain.

Characteristics of Optimum Criteria and Tests

Given that death is the permanent cessation of functioning of the organism as a whole, a criterion or set of tests will yield a false positive if it incorrectly denies the possibility for that organism to function as a whole. By far the most important requirement for a criterion of death and for a test is to yield no false positives.

Of secondary importance, the criterion and tests should produce few and relatively brief false negatives, such as the prediction that the organism as a whole may again function when it will not. Current tests may produce many false negatives during the thirty-minute to twenty-four-hour interval between the successive neurologic examinations required for the determination of irreversible whole brain dysfunction. Certain sets of tests, particularly those requiring electrocerebral silence by EEG, may produce false negative determinations if EEG artifact is present and cannot confidently be distinguished from brain wave activity. Generally, a few brief false negatives are tolerable and even inevitable, since tests must be delineated conservatively in order to eliminate any possibility of false positives.

Further, as has been noted,[10] every physician should be able to use the tests easily to determine that the criterion is satisfied. Also, although the tests are established, validated, applied, and interpreted by medical professionals, they must originate in a criterion with significance understandable to a layperson.

Permanent Loss of Cardiopulmonary Functioning

The permanent termination of heart and lung function has been a criterion of death throughout history. The ancients observed that all other bodily functions ceased shortly after cessation of these vital functions, and the irreversible process of bodily disintegration inevitably followed. Thus, loss of spontaneous cardiopulmonary function was found to predict permanent nonfunctioning of the organism as a whole, therefore serving adequately as a criterion of death.

Because of current ventilation/perfusion technology, the loss of spontaneous cardiopulmonary functioning is no longer necessarily a prediction of permanent nonfunctioning of the organism as a whole. To consider a conscious talking patient with apnea from bulbar poliomyelitis requiring an iron lung and who has developed asystole requiring a permanent pacemaker as dead is absurd.

Also, now that ventilation and perfusion can be mechanically maintained, an organism with permanent loss of whole brain functioning can have permanently ceased to function as a whole days to weeks before the heart and lungs cease to function with artificial support. In this light, the heart and lungs seem to have no special relationship to the functioning of the organism as a whole. Continued artificially supported cardiopulmonary function is no longer perfectly correlated with life and the loss of spontaneous cardiopulmonary functioning is no longer perfectly correlated with death.

Total and Irreversible Loss of Whole
Brain Functioning

The criterion for cessation of functioning of the organism as a whole is permanent loss of functioning of the entire brain. This criterion is perfectly correlated with the permanent cessation of functioning of the organism as a whole because the brain is necessary for the functioning of the organism as a whole. It integrates, generates, interrelates, and controls complex bodily activities. A patient on a ventilator with a totally destroyed brain is merely a group of artificially maintained subsystems since the organism as a whole has ceased to function. Korein[11] has made a further defense of the brain as the critical system controlling the organism as a whole, using thermodynamics and information theory.

The brain generates the signal for breathing through brainstem ventilatory centers, and aids in the control of circulation through medullary blood pressure control centers. Destruction of the brain produces apnea and generalized vasodilatation; in all cases, despite the most aggressive support, the adult heart stops within one week, and that of the child within two weeks.[12] Thus, when the organism as a whole has ceased to function, the artificially supported "vital" subsystems quickly fail. Many other functions of the organism as a whole, including neuroendocrine control, temperature control, food searching behaviors, and sexual activity, reside in the more primitive regions (hypothalamus, brainstem) of the brain. Thus total and irreversible loss of funtioning of the whole brain and not merely the neocortex is required as the criterion for the permanent loss of the functioning of the organism as a whole.

Using permanent loss of functioning of the whole brain as the criterion for death of the organism as a whole is also consistent with tradition. Throughout history, whenever a physician was called to ascertain the occurrence of death, the examination importantly

included the following signs indicative of permanent loss of functioning of the whole brain: unresponsivity, lack of spontaneous movements including breathing, and absence of pupillary light response.
Only one important sign, lack of heartbeat, was not directly indicative of whole brain destruction. Yet the heartbeat stops within several minutes of apnea and permanent absence of the "vital signs" is
an important sign of permanent loss of whole brain functioning.
Thus, permanent loss of whole brain functioning has in an important
sense always been the underlying criterion of death.

THE TESTS OF DEATH

Given the definition of death as the permanent cessation of functioning of the organism as a whole, and the criterion of death as the total
and irreversible cessation of functioning of the whole brain, the next
step is examination of the available tests of death.

Cessation of Heartbeat and Ventilation

The physical findings of permanent absence of heartbeat and respira-
tion are the traditional tests of death. In the vast majority of deaths
not complicated by artificial ventilation, these classic tests are still
applicable. They show that the criterion of death has been satisfied
since they always quickly produce permanent loss of functioning of
the whole brain. However, when mechanical ventilation is being used,
these tests lose most of their utility due to the production of numerous false negatives for as long a time as days to weeks, for example,
death of the organism as a whole with still intact circulatory-ventilatory subsystems. Thus determination of the circulation-ventilation
tests will suffice in most instances of death, and only in the case of
artificial maintenance of circulation or ventilation will the special
brain dysfunction tests be needed.

Irreversible Cessation of Whole Brain Functioning

Numerous formalized sets of tests have been established to determine
that the criterion of permanent loss of whole brain functioning has

been met. These include, among others, the publications of the Harvard Medical School Ad Hoc Committee[13] and the National Institutes of Health Collaborative Study of Cerebral Survival.[14] They all have been recently reviewed.[15, 16] What we call tests have sometimes themselves been called "criteria," but it is important to distinguish these second-level criteria from the first-level criteria. While the first-level criteria determining the death of an organism must be understood by the layperson, the second-level criteria or tests determining permanent loss of functioning of the whole brain need not be understood by anyone except qualified clinicians. To avoid confusion, we prefer to use the designation tests for the second-level criteria.

All the proposed tests require total and permanent absence of all functioning of the brainstem and both hemispheres. They vary slightly from one set to another, but all require unresponsivity (deep coma), absent pupillary light reflexes, apnea, and absent cephalic reflexes, including corneals, gag, oculovestibulars, and oculocephalics. They also require the absence of drug intoxication, and the newer sets require the demonstration of a structural brain lesion. Isoelectrical EEGs are generally required, and tests disclosing absence of cerebral blood flow are of confirmatory value.[17] All tests require the given dysfunction to be present for a particular time interval, which in the case of absence of cerebral blood flow may be as short as thirty minutes.

There are ample studies (reviewed by Vcith and associates[18] that show perfect correlation between the brain dysfunction tests of the Ad Hoc Committee of the Harvard Medical School and total brain necrosis at postmortem examination. Veith and associates[19] conclude that "the validity of the criteria must be considered to be established with as much certainty as is possible in biology or medicine." Thus, when a physician ascertains that a patient fulfills the validated brain dysfunction tests, he or she can be confident that the loss of whole brain functioning is permanent. Physicians should only apply tests which have been completed validated.

THE DETERMINATION OF DEATH

The consideration of several examples of death to illustrate the applications of our analysis is helpful. We will review deaths by primary respiratory arrest, primary cardiac arrest, and primary brain destruction. In each case the process of dying, the event of death, and the process of disintegration will be identified.

Death by Hanging: In a properly executed hanging, a displaced fracture of the odontoid process ("hangman's fracture") occurs that acutely compresses the cervical spinal cord and produces instantaneous apnea. Some degree of airway compromise and carotid artery compression undoubtedly also occurs, but we will restrict our attention to the principal fatal effect, that of primary respiratory arrest.

As apnea persists, progressive hypoxemia and acidosis produce cardiac arrest within several minutes. Throughout this time, the brain is becoming progressively ischemic and finally, within a short period after cardiac arrest, suffers total infarction. Cooling, lividity, and rigor mortis inevitably follow.

Although stating that death occurs at the moment of the neck fracture may sound plausible, clearly this is not the case. The neck fracture and subsequent respiratory and cardiac arrests are part of the process of dying. Only once the whole brain has become irreversibly dysfunctional by the cardiopulmonary arrest has the event of death occurred. This event is then followed by the process of disintegration. If the victim had been placed on a ventilator immediately after the neck fracture, permanent loss of whole brain functioning would have been prevented. Thus the process of dying would have been reversed and death prevented. A similar, and even more dramatic example, is death by decapitation, though at present there may be no way to reverse this process.

Death by Chronic Disease: Many patients dying of chronic diseases suffer spontaneous ventricular fibrillation. As cardiac output ceases, so does cerebral blood flow so that the brain becomes progressively ischemic. When medullary ischemia occurs, apnea is produced, which accelerates the loss of brain and other organ functioning. Finally the brain becomes totally infarcted, and events of disintegration proceed.

Although ventricular fibrillation may be said to be the proximal cause of death, clearly the patient is not dead at the moment the heart stops or even at the time the respirations cease. At these times the patient is dying. Death occurs when the brain has become totally and irreversibly dysfunctional by ischemic infarction. A timely resuscitation prior to total loss of brain functioning would reverse the process of dying. Death, of course, is irreversible by definition.

Death by Massive Head Injury: These injuries are often complicated by immediate and severe cerebral edema. When the resulting increased intracranial pressure exceeds that of systolic blood pressure, cerebral blood flow ceases and whole brain infarction occurs. At the time of head injury or minutes later when whole brain infarction is proceeding, medullary failure produces apnea. Progressive hypoxemia and acidosis then produce ventricular fibrillation or asystole. Untreated, the organism undergoes the process of cooling, dependent lividity, and rigor mortis.

However, if the patient were placed on a ventilator immediately after irreversible whole brain dysfunction but prior to cardiac arrest, the circulatory functioning could probably be maintained for a few days. If bedside testing confirmed fulfillment of validated brain dysfunction tests, the difficult situation of preserved circulatory-ventilatory subsystems despite the cessation of functioning of the organism as a whole would be present. Death would have occurred at the time the brain had totally and permanently lost all functioning. In this case, mechanical ventilation and other aggressive therapeutics would have delayed the process of disintegration, although the event of death has already occurred.

THE STATUTE OF DEATH

Veith and colleagues[20] have recently emphasized the need for recognizing the role of the brain in determining death in statutory definitions of death. The model statute of Capron and Kass, the best-known and adopted by five states, reads:

> A person will be considered dead if in the announced opinion of a physician, based on ordinary standards of medical practice, he has experienced an irreversible cessation of spontaneous respiratory and circulatory functions. In the event that artificial means of support preclude a determination that these functions have ceased, a person will be considered dead if in the announced opinion of a physician, based on ordinary standards of medical practice, he has experienced an irreversible cessation of spontaneous brain functions. Death will have occurred at the time when the relevant functions ceased.[21]

The Capron–Kass statute, like the Kansas statute[22] that it criticizes, has two distinct criteria: first, irreversible cessation of spontaneous respiratory and circulatory functions; and second, when this cannot be determined, irreversible cessation of spontaneous brain functions. No explanation is given for the reason irreversible cessation of spontaneous brain functions should be used only when one cannot determine that the other criterion is satisfied. And indeed, there is no reason for limiting its use in that way. If someone's head is cut off or completely crushed, there is no need to determine that the person has also suffered an irreversible cessation of spontaneous respiratory and circulatory functions.

Recognizing that the Capron–Kass statute had two distinct criteria, in 1975 the American Bar Association (A.B.A.) published their model statute of death.[23] It states: "For all legal purposes, a human body with irreversible cessation of total brain function, according to usual and customary standards of medical practice, shall be considered dead."

Because this statute has a single criterion of death, the irreversible cessation of whole brain functioning, it is an improvement over that of Capron–Kass. However, it has a shortcoming which Capron and Kass have avoided. It does not state that physicians can declare death in their customary fashion, using the circulation-ventilation tests in the overwhelming majority of deaths not complicated by artificial ventilation.

We propose a statute with a single criterion that does not require any change in current medical practice. It states:

> A person will be considered dead if in the announced opinion of a physician, based on ordinary standards of medical practice, he has experienced an irreversible cessation of all brain functions. Irreversible cessation of spontaneous respiratory and circulatory functions shall be considered sufficient proof for the irreversible cessation of brain functions in the absence of any medical evidence to the contrary. Death will have occurred at the time when the brain functions have irreversibly ceased.[24]

This statute has several advantages over the Capron–Kass proposal. First, it meets all of the standards that they proposed for an acceptable statute. It does not result in Brierley's patients being declared dead. Indeed, all and only those patients determined to be dead by the Capron–Kass statute meet the criterion of this statute. Thus it allows for the change in the declaration of death they desire, without going too far. It is incremental, but unlike their statutory definition, it proposes a single criterion. Irreversible cessation of whole brain functioning is the criterion of death. Additionally, this statute allows physicians to make their determinations of death in exactly the way they do now, which is an improvement over the A.B.A. statute.

By using the irreversible cessation of spontaneous circulatory and respiratory functions as a test for irreversible loss of whole brain function, our proposed statute allows us to answer the question raised by Jonas:[25] "Why are they alive if the heart, etc., works naturally but not alive when it works artificially?" Spontaneous circulation and ventilation proves that at least part of the brain continues to function whereas artificial support does not show this. Thus in the latter case one needs to discover directly if the whole brain has permanently ceased to function.

Finally, our statute explicitly states the fact that it is the brain, not the heart and lungs, that is important in the functioning of the organism as a whole. Thus it allows for new technological advances, such as a totally implantable artificial heart that may continue to function after the brain has ceased to function.

In conclusion, we include only what we really believe to be the criterion for death in our statutory definition: the irreversible cessation of total brain functions. We use irreversible cessation of spontaneous ventilation and circulation as the usual method for determining death, as the Capron and Kass statute prescribes, but unlike them, we do not elevate this method into a criterion of death. Rather, it is considered as presently used, the most common test for determining that the criterion of death—irreversible total cessation of whole brain functioning—has been satisfied.

NOTES TO CHAPTER 10

1.   R.S. Morison, "Death: Process or Event?," *Science* 173 (1971): 694–8.
2.   B. Gert, "Can the Brain Have Pain?," *Philosophy and Phenomenological Research* 27 (1967): 432–6.
3.   B. Gert, "Personal Identity and the Body," *Dialogue* 10 (1971): 458–78.
4.   G. Grisez and J.M. Boyle, Jr., *Life and Death with Liberty and Justice: A Contribution to the Euthanasia Debate* (Notre Dame, Indiana: University of Notre Dame Press, 1979).
5.   R.M. Veatch, *Death, Dying and the Biological Revolution: Our Last Quest for Responsibility* (New Haven: Yale University Press, 1976).
6.   H.R. Beresford, "The Quinlan Decision: Problems and Legislative Alternatives," *Annals of Neurology* 2 (1977): 74–81.
7.   J.B. Brierley, et al., "Neocortical Death After Cardiac Arrest," *Lancet* 2 (1975): 560–5.

8. B. Jennett and F. Plum, "Persistent Vegetative State After Brain Damage: A Syndrome in Search of a Name," *Lancet* 1 (1972): 734-7.

9. Veatch, "Death, Dying, and the Biological Revolution."

10. Task Force on Death and Dying of the Institute of Society, Ethics, and the Life Sciences, "Refinements in Criteria for the Determination of Death: An Appraisal," *Journal of the American Medical Association* 221 (1972): 48-53.

11. J. Korein, "The Problem of Brain Death," *Annals of the New York Academy of Sciences* 315 (1978): 19-38.

12. D.H. Ingvar, et al., "Survival After Severe Cerebral Anoxia with Destruction of the Cerebral Cortex: the Apallic Syndrome," *Annals of the New York Academy of Sciences* 315 (1978): 184-214.

13. H.K. Beecher, "A Definition of Irreversible Coma: Report of the Ad Hoc Committee of the Harvard Medical School to Examine the Definition of Brain Death," *Journal of the American Medical Association* 205 (1968): 337-40.

14. "An Appraisal of the Criteria of Cerebral Death: A Summary Statement," *Journal of the American Medical Association* 237 (1977): 982-6.

15. P.M. Black, "Brain Death," *New England Journal of Medicine* 299 (1978): 338-44, 393-401.

16. G.F. Molinari, "Review of Clinical Criteria of Brain Death," *Annals of New York Academy of Sciences* 315 (1978): 62-9.

17. "An Appraisal of the Criteria of Cerebral Death," op. cit.

18. F.J. Veith, et al., "Brain Death: I. A Status Report of Medical and Ethical Considerations," *Journal of the American Medical Association* 238 (1977): 1651-5.

19. *Ibid.*

20. *Ibid.*

21. A.M. Capron and L.R. Kass, "A Statutory Definition of the Standards for Determining Human Death: An Appraisal and a Proposal," *University of Pennsylvania Law Review* 121 (1972): 87-118.

22. I.M. Kennedy, "The Kansas Statute on Death—An Appraisal," *New England Journal of Medicine* 285 (1971): 946-50.

23. "House of Delegates Redefines Death, Urges Redefinition of Rape, and Undoes the Houston Amendments," *American Bar Association Journal* 61 (1975): 463-4.

24. In a more recent paper, the authors argue for a statute defining death that they believe is preferable to the statute in the text above. That statute is:

    An individual who has sustained irreversible cessation of all functions of the entire brain, including the brainstem, is dead.
    (a) In the absence of artificial means of cardiopulmonary support, death (the irreversible cessation of all brain functions) may be determined by the prolonged absence of spontaneous circulatory and respiratory functions.

(b) In the presence of artificial means of cardiopulmonary support, death (the irreversible cessation of all brain functions) must be determined by tests of brain function.

In both situations, the determination of death must be made in accordance with accepted medical standards. See Bernat, Culver, and Gert, "Defining Death in Theory and Practice," *The Hastings Center Report* 12 (1982): pp. 5–9.

25.   H. Jonas, *Philosophical Essays: From Ancient Creed to Technological Man* (Englewood Cliffs, New Jersey: Prentice-Hall, 1974), pp. 134–40.

11 WHEN TO KEEP PATIENTS ALIVE AGAINST THEIR WISHES

Bart Gruzalski

"Donald was admitted in a critical but conscious state. He sustained second and third-degree burns over sixty-eight percent of his body—mostly third degree burns. Both eyes were blinded by corneal damage. . . . On one occasion Donald put the matter very bluntly: 'What gives a physician the right to keep alive a patient who wants to die?' " Case No. 228, *Hastings Center Report*, June, 1975.

There are cases in which it would be wrong to keep a person alive against his or her wishes, and other cases in which such an act is obligatory. It would be wrong to treat a person against his or her wishes in the following case: a patient's life could be prolonged a few days by use of a painful protocol, but the patient explicitly wants to die more quickly and more peacefully without the debilitating treatment. The following is an example of when it would be right to treat a person against his or her wishes: a car accident victim has witnessed the death of the others in the car, is in shock, and is refusing treatment but needs emergency care to prevent bleeding to death. Between these relatively noncontroversial cases lies a range of controversial cases involving badly injured patients who can be kept alive with medical intervention but who, at least for a time, say that they do not want life-saving treatment.

The specific controversial cases on which I focus in this chapter are severe burn victims and persons with cervical spinal cord injuries who have refused or are refusing any life-prolonging (as opposed to palliative) medical care. These cases often exhibit overt conflicts of value for, while the victim is explicitly making a choice that presupposes his or her life is not worth living, the members of the medical staff may want to act in ways which presuppose that the patient's life is worth living. This value conflict not only causes suffering for the patient, but also makes it difficult for members of the medical team to be comfortable either honoring the patient's wishes or doing what they believe to be in the best interests of the patient. Underlying some of this tension is the nagging question: When is it morally permissible to keep burn victims and spinal cord patients alive against their wishes, and when is it not? Our discussion will provide a basis for what will permit us to answer this question decisively in at least some cases, so that as far as possible we may avoid acting on the basis of unexamined convention and also avoid imposing our values on those who do not share them.

A PRIMA FACIE JUSTIFICATION OF PATERNALISTIC INTERVENTION

To treat a person against his or her expressed choice is a violation of liberty.[1] But when a person is incompetent due to drugs, stress, grief, or related debilitating factors, we sometimes believe that we must overrule a person's liberty for his or her own good. In this chapter we focus upon persons who are experiencing just such incapacitating conditions: the two types of seriously injured patients in question suffer from shock, grief, pain, depression, and the psychological effects of powerful drugs, and find themselves in medical facilities that are able to keep them alive against their wishes. These conditions make it nearly impossible for such persons to make fully rational choices. For instance, a severely depressed person may be simply unable to assess his or her future and, hence, be unable to make a rational choice involving alternative actions that will lead to different futures. In addition, the patient in an acute phase is "trapped" in a very special environment, has been separated from his or her primary group, has perhaps barely escaped death, may have witnessed the deaths of others, and is often angry, depressed and distrustful of caretakers.[2] Finally, even though such patients may refuse treatments, after their wishes are overridden they often come to be grateful for the treatment they wanted to reject. Such patients are not noncontroversially competent to make life and death decisions for themselves and, so, are prime candidates for paternalistic interventions: interventions for what the invervening persons believe to be the patient's own good but against the patient's wishes.[3] Although a patient may be a candidate for such intervention, that does not automatically justify contravening the patient's wishes.

TWO STRATEGIES OF PATERNALISTIC INTERVENTION FOR BADLY INJURED PATIENTS

In this section we will examine two strategies of paternalistic intervention for badly injured patients. The first I refer to as the "life-maintenance strategy." According to this strategy, we should keep severely injured patients alive both because and until they can later assess the value of their lives and act accordingly. The second strategy is the "case-by-case strategy": the caretaker, the psychiatric consultant, and the appropriate ethics committee members review each case and evaluate it on its own merits. Let's begin by discussing the life-maintenance strategy for badly injured patients.

The point of the "life-maintenance strategy" is to try to keep the patient alive if there are chances of survival.[4] The rationale for doing this begins with the fact that the patient may be suffering from shock, may be grieving the loss of bodily functions, may be grieving over the corresponding loss of social abilities, is likely in a stressful environment, is likely in pain, and may also be under the influence of powerful psychophysical drugs. Any patient in these conditions is under enough duress that there is *prima facie* evidence for thinking that such a patient is incompetent to make a rational choice. Since this would not be sufficient justification to keep such a patient alive, the rationale for treatment requires the further argument that if the patient is kept alive, then later, when not under such duress, the patient can decide upon the course of treatment—including suicide. This strategy allows us to avoid one kind of "worst case scenario," viz., allowing the patient to die when the patient would later have been grateful to have been kept alive. In summary, this first strategy in cases involving badly injured persons is defended on the grounds that treatment "would make possible his (the patient's) further deliberation on whether he wished to live."[5]

The point of the "case-by-case strategy," on the other hand, is to treat each patient as unique and to decide each case on its individual merits. One problem with this approach is that by emphasizing the uniqueness of patients, we may overlook that what justifies a line of action for one patient justifies the same line of action for a relevantly similar patient. A closely related problem is that this approach does not explicitly recognize any grounds on which we may determine whether a treatment decision is correct. For this reason it is hard to see how the case-by-case approach does not simply fluctuate between a deference to liberty and a deference to the view that any life, however horrid, is worth living. For example, H. Tristram Engelhardt, in commenting on the burn case referred to in the opening quote of this chapter, claims that:

> when the patient decides that the future quality of life open to him is not worth the investment of pain and suffering to attain that future quality of life, that is a decision proper to the patient . . . *one must be willing, as a price for recognizing the freedom of others, to live with the consequences of that freedom: some persons will make choices that they would regret were they to live longer* [italics mine].[6]

But contrast Engelhardt's opinion with that of Arthur Dyck, Professor of Population Ethics at Harvard School of Public Health and Harvard Divinity School:

> The courage to be, as expressed in Christian and Jewish thought, is more than the overcoming of the fear of death, although it includes that stoic dimension. It is the courage to accept one's own life as having worth *no matter what life may bring*, including the threat of death, because that life remains meaningful and is regarded as worthy of God, *regardless of what that life may be like*. . . . Suffering does not render a life meaningless or worthless. Suffering people need the support of others; suffering people should not be encouraged to commit suicide by their community, or that community ceases to be a community [italics mine].[7]

Obviously, it would make a great deal of difference to a badly injured patient whether he or she were in a unit that looked to an Engelhardt or to a Dyck for ethical guidance.

To make matters even worse, unless a decision about how to proceed in such a case is grounded on some relatively clear rationale, it may be only the product of that day's psychological outlook of the care provider, psychiatrist, hospital counsel, judge, or Institutional Review Board member whose opinion became decisive. We all know that there are days during which life seems worth living despite tremendous physical, social, or economic setbacks, as well as days during which life barely seems worth living in the midst of what would typically be considered fortunate circumstances. Such psychological states cannot but affect the outcome of a concerned and caring assessment of the difficult cases in question. Thus it is crucial to ask whether there are any objective grounds for deciding such cases— grounds that are not determined by the fears, moods, religious convictions, or other features of the decisionmakers that do not reflect the attitudes and preferences of the victim. Because the case-by-case strategy is of itself empty of content, it may lull care providers, however well-intentioned they may be, into acting on the basis of values not shared by the patient.

THE CONTRIBUTION OF ETHICAL THEORY

In assessing the moral rightness and wrongness of actions, we find two fundamental ethical views that not only explain many of our thought-out moral judgments, but also express underlying intuitions about the nature of morality. One of these views is based on respect for persons and finds its classical statement in the writings of Immanuel Kant: "Act so that you treat humanity, whether in your own person or that of another, always as an end and never as a means only."[8] In this version of his categorical imperative, Kant is *not* making the impossible demand that we should *never* use any person as a means to an end. Rather, what he is saying is that one should not *only* or *merely* treat another person as a device or as a "means." One standard interpretation of this imperative is that we should not force another to do anything against his or her will. As one philosopher recently wrote: "Individuals are ends and not merely means; they may not be sacrificed or used for the achieving of other ends without their consent."[9]

Since the kind of intervention on which we are focusing involves treating patients *against* their wishes, the Kantian view poses a prima facie argument against our doing so. Although there is a strong prima facie case here, to pretend that this conclusion characterizes the Kantian view in our cases would be shortsighted. First, it is not clear, for precisely the reasons that make these cases troublesome, what is the person's will. Patients in the acute phase may be disoriented, delusional, in pain, fearful, and incoherent—in short, suffering from those conditions that are among the constituents of psychological coercion and, hence, are taken to undermine or contravene a person's will. In addition, such stress often incapacitates persons so that they are unable to assess the future and their corresponding options. In any such case the person's explicit *wish* may violate the person's *will* because the person is underinformed.[10] For example, a depressed person may attempt to commit suicide because of the false belief that the future holds no opportunities for him or her.[11] Yet if we are confident that the person's assessment of the future is unrealistic and is only a temporary condition resulting from depression, we may act in a way that is consistent with the settled values and preferences that characterize the person's autonomous self. To fail to act in such a way is to pretend *either* that persons are not vulnerable to depressions and other duress which might cause them to act contrary to their own deepest values, *or* that a self-destructive wish caused by a temporary depression is as much an expression of the person's will as any other value which might characterize the person or to which the person might be committed. Since both claims are often false, it follows even on Kantian grounds that we ought, in some cases, to act on the behalf of a patient against his or her expressed wishes.

The second fundamental view of morality focuses on the results of one's actions: A person ought to perform actions likely to promote the happiness of everyone affected by the actions and, hence, no one should perform actions likely to produce unnecessary pain and suffering.[12] John Stuart Mill, in articulating this view, "holds that actions are right in proportion as they tend to promote happiness; wrong as they tend to produce the reverse of happiness."[13] By 'happiness' Mill means "pleasure and the absence of pain," and by 'unhappiness', "pain and the privation of pleasure." Furthermore, "As between his own happiness and that of others, utilitarianism requires him (any agent) to be as strictly impartial as a disinterested and benevolent spectator."

In order more easily to examine what the utilitarian would say in cases of badly injured patients, and because the positive effects of keeping alive or allowing to die will likely cancel out the negative effects on third parties (family, staff, and so on), we will omit any consideration of these effects of intervening on third parties. Instead, we only consider the effects that intervening may have on the patient. It may be thought that to assess the effects of the action on the patient a utilitarian need not take into account the patient's expressed wishes. But this is false. A person's expressed wishes are one important datum of evidence for what that person will likely value and find to be either a source of happiness or a source of suffering. Furthermore, to frustrate a person's expressed wishes is itself an excellent way to cause suffering, at least in the short term. On the other hand, it is true that people often wish what would not, in fact, bring them happiness. Persons in acute stages who are in shock, in pain, and beginning to grieve over the loss of physical aspects of themselves are as likely as anyone to fail to foresee what might bring them happiness in the long run. Hence, although a patient's expressed wishes are some evidence for what will benefit the patient in the long run, we must conclude that in our cases this evidence becomes tenuous.

THE REVIEW OF THE LIFE-MAINTENANCE STRATEGY

Having briefly examined the two basic ethical views that serve as the general bases for evaluating actions, let us apply these views to the strategy of keeping all such patients alive as long as they are in an acute phase. On the surface, each view seems to support such a strategy. Consider the Kantian position. Insofar as we are showing respect for persons and trying to respect the victim's deepest will, keeping every such patient alive may be seen as a way of doing what we can to permit the person's will to function as fully as it is able in the following sense: After the acute phase is passed (during which the patient's will is affected by stress, pain, and anxiety), the patient is in a position to express and carry out his or her will. If at that point the patient no longer wills to stay alive, the patient can terminate life-prolonging treatments or, if necessary, commit suicide. A similar rationale seems to emerge from the utilitarian position. Once the acute phase is passed and the victim is no longer reacting from stress and pain, the patient alone has the privileged inner access to decide whether life is happy enough to make it worth living. If the balance of suffering outweighs whatever is positive, then the patient will know it and will also be in a position either to terminate life-prolonging treatment or to commit suicide.

There is, however, a deep conceptual reason why both the person-respecting and the suffering-minimizing ethical views condemn the simplistic life-maintenance strategy. The best way to bring this out is to contrast the following two evaluations:

1. My life is (now) worth living; and
2. It was worth the pain and stress of treatment to keep me alive to this point.

It is important to see that a person can affirm the first evaluation while denying the second. A person may affirm that staying alive is now "worth it," but that it was not worth the pain and suffering to reach this state. For example, a severely burned man may say that his life is worth living after he's been somewhat rehabilitated—he is alive *and at this point* it would not be worth either killing himself or omitting some life-saving treatment. Yet the same patient may *also* say that the pain, anxiety, and stress he had to suffer to reach this point far outweigh the positive aspects of now being alive. Two non-medical examples may further clarify how the two evaluations differ. Suppose a couple in their eighties agree that their relationship is now worth maintaining: there is no point to their breaking up and, in fact, they have grown accustomed to each other. Nonetheless, the same persons may also agree that forty years ago it would have been wise to end the relationship and that the payoff of forty years of un-happy marriage—a bit of security in old age—was not worth the forty years of strife. In this nonmedical example the two people affirm an analogue of the first evaluation, viz., that their marriage is now worth maintaining. But they are *also* affirming the negation of the analogue of the second evaluation, viz., that some security in old age does not make forty years of unhappy marriage worth it. Or, suppose you skip a movie to go to a cocktail party. You may agree that, since you're there, it is worth being there [the analogue of (1)], but it wasn't worth the sacrifice [denying the analogue of (2)].

If we apply this distinction to the life-maintenance strategy, we see how this strategy is condemned on both Kantian and utilitarian ethical accounts. Even though the patient, after the acute stage, may affirm that life is now worth living, he may *still* wish that we had not made him undergo the paternalistic intervention and condemn us for having made the wrong decision. This response shows, as far as any response can, that we have violated the patient's deepest will as it was (or would have been) at the time of our intervention. Hence, not only is keeping *all* badly injured persons alive not a good method for satisfying the Kantian person-respecting ethic, but such a strategy is not even justified should the person agree that his or her life is subsequently worth living [that is, affirm (1)]. The crucial question is whether the patient has come to welcome the intervention (to *affirm* that the intervention was worth it). A similar observation shows that utilitarianism does not justify the life-maintenance strategy in these cases. A person may agree that, from this point on, there will probably be more happiness than suffering in his or her life, and for that reason it would be irrational to commit suicide now. But the same person may also say that it would have been better to have been allowed to die because no foreseeable amount of happiness could balance out the amount of suffering sustained since the point of injury. Hence, from a utilitarian point of view, the decision to keep the person alive causes more foreseeable suffering than happiness, and so is wrong.

In addition to this conceptual reason for abandoning the life-maintenance strategy in cases of severe bodily injury, there are profoundly humane reasons to do so. A patient may not only affirm that the intervention was not worth it [thus denying (2) above], but may also affirm that life is now not worth living [denying (1)]. Nonetheless a person may not be psychologically able or willing to terminate even "ordinary" treatment, much less to commit suicide. For example, were the patient a staunch Roman Catholic, that person would not commit suicide even if life had become only a prolonged agony. On the other hand, were a patient to commit suicide, we would have forced the patient through a terribly painful and tragically unnecessary ordeal.

THE RATIONALE FOR A MORE OBJECTIVE STRATEGY

On the basis of our discussion we may draw out two criteria that must be satisfied if a paternalistic intervention is to be justified. The first is:

A. The patient is not fully competent to assess what will happen if he or she is treated, what will happen if he or she is not treated, and which results are better.

Assuming that we are able to apply (A) with some degree of reliability, it is clear that the satisfaction of (A) would not of itself justify a paternalistic treatment. For example, it would be wrong to override the refusal of an othodox and practicing Jehovah's Witness who was clear about wanting "no blood" but who also was in shock and, hence, not fully competent. It would also be wrong to force a terminal cancer patient through a last round of tests that he or she did not want, even though the patient was not clear about the point of the tests (perhaps to discover a way of prolonging life a few days) but was adamant about wanting to be allowed to "die in peace." Because (A) is satisfied in each of these cases, it follows that the satisfaction of (A) is not enough to justify a paternalistic treatment. At best, (A) is only a necessary condition of paternalistic action, although there are even difficulties with treating (A) as a necessary condition. For example, a paranoid schizophrenic with an adequately high IQ and a good academic education may be able to converse intelligently and even insightfully for a limited period of time in a protected environment and, for this reason, may seem to be competent. On the other hand, a less educated person who is accustomed to communicating with his or her body may simply say and then act out what is, in fact, the refusal of an adequately competent person. Finally, there is always the danger that a person who claims to want to die will be labelled "irrational" by caretakers who would not themselves want to die in the patient's circumstances.[14]

In short, it is not only *not* true that some degree of mental incompetency is reason enough to keep a patient alive against the patient's wishes, it is often unclear when a person is incompetent to make important decisions. Although these observations raise the troublesome question of whether or not we are justified in treating (A) as a necessary condition of paternalistic actions, two considerations will show that (A) is satisfied in the cases with which we are concerned. The first is that severe burn victims and cervical spinal cord injury patients are typically in pain, shock, often delusional, experiencing grief, or under the stress of being in a new environment in which they have practically no control, not even over the fate of their own bodies. Second, such patients often later welcome our intervention, which suggests that something was amiss with their earlier wish to die, even from their own point of view.

This second observation points to a central criterion that we must satisfy if we are to justify intervening in such cases. The second criterion expresses the requirement that paternalistic interventions correspond as far as possible to the person's own assessment of the positive and negative results of the intervention by reflecting the deeper will of the person which would express itself were the person not under duress. This second criterion helps us to identify what the person would, if not incompetent, see as being in his or her best interests. Hence, if satisfied, it would seem to justify treating incompetent patients against their wishes:

B. The person will come to welcome the intervention.

We have good reasons for thinking that (B) is a sufficient condition for intervening in the case of the incompetent patient. When (B) applies we have evidence for claiming that the person was incompetent [viz., that (A) applies]. But more importantly, when (B) applies it reflects both the Kantian and the utilitarian moral views discussed above. If the person says that we did what the patient would have willed had he or she known enough and been able to assess clearly the pain, grief, and anxiety, what more could be asked by a Kantian as evidence that the intervention reflected the victim's deeper will? If the patient says that the suffering was worth it and is outweighed by the happiness or pleasures that followed, what else could a utilitarian demand insofar as the utilitarian is assessing the happiness or suffering of the patient that will result from a decision to treat?[15]

Of course, more might be available: "living wills" and similar documents that request or refuse treatment in just such cases. But what if these documents were inconsistent with (B)? There are two plausible explanations for such an inconsistency. The first is that the patient is now better informed about the alternatives than he or she was when making out the "living will." This possibility brings out one serious problem with such a document: the "cool moment" reflection of a person in his or her study, kitchen, or lawyer's office may not reflect an adequate appreciation of the alternatives that the badly injured patient confronts. This specific problem with prior expressions of choice in life and death matters was recently cited by Seattle internist Dr. Norman K. Brown: "You can pass living wills around a roomful of young people and 95 percent will sign them. . . . But pass them around a nursing home and you'll get a different response."[16] The discrepancy Dr. Brown cites is just the sort that could well occur when comparing the less informed wishes of the healthy with the better informed assessments of those badly injured patients who are no longer under the duress experienced in the more acute phase of their injuries.

The second reason a "living will" may be inconsistent with a subsequent welcoming of the paternalistic treatment is that the treatment itself *caused* the patient to be unable not to welcome it. The starkest case would be one in which a person's brain is so reconstructed that the person is caused to welcome the reconstruction.[17] Although such a case is currently a technical impossibility, it is worth exploring what would be objectional about producing a situation that *causes* the patient to consent. It is *not* that the favorable consent is predictable, since that will be true of the cases best justified on paternalistic grounds. (For example, a man who unwittingly consumes LSD and, as a result of his altered state, prepares to launch himself off the edge of a five-story apartment building for a flight over Boston will predictably come to welcome a timely intervention.) Rather, the difficulty is that the brain reconstruction patient *cannot do* otherwise. In making the patient's subsequent rejection physically or psychologically impossible, we have removed the possibility of choice and assessment, and that is what is offensive about the imagined brain reconstruction. Significantly, this explanation of our moral repugnance at such an intervention corresponds with the inadequacy of such a justification from both the Kantian and the utilitarian points of view. From a Kantian point of view, the person's will has been altered and hence the subsequent affirmation does not express the person's deeper will *at the time of treatment.* From the utilitarian point of view, the person *is not able to assess* the merits of the intervention and, hence, any postoperative assessments are without value. It follows that such an intervention, even though satisfying (B), would not be justified, and, hence, a requirement in addition to (B) is needed.

C. If (B) is satisfied, that is, if the patient comes to welcome the intervention, it must be the case that the patient was able to assess the intervention negatively.[18]

Although we would not be justified in intervening in cases unless (C) is satisfied in addition to (B), it is difficult to find cases that are ruled out by (C). The imaginary brain reconstruction case is one, and, perhaps, examples involving posthypnotic suggestion would constitute others. But in the cases on which we are focusing, the subsequent welcomings, if any, are not caused in this way. If the burn victim or the quadraplegic is subsequently glad to be alive, there is no good reason to believe that the "will" of the person has been coerced or that the person is unable to make an assessment of what has happened. These ex-patients *can* judge that the interventions should not have been performed. Hence, we may use (A), (B) and (C) to assess life-saving paternalistic interventions for burn patients or paralyzed patients who have been recently injured.

TWO TEST CASES

It will be useful to test these criteria by applying them to the following cases:

Case 1: A 25 year old married woman was admitted to a hospital having lost two-thirds of her body's blood supply from a ruptured ulcer. The woman and her husband, both Jehovah's Witnesses, had signed a document releasing the physician and the hospital from any liability that might result from the failure to administer blood. Both the husband and the wife refused to approve a blood transfusion.[19]

Case 2: A 52 year old married man was admitted semi-conscious to an intensive care unit after a suicide attempt. He had adapted to his multiple sclerosis, which had been the cause of progressive physical disability over a fifteen-year period. Three weeks prior to the suicide attempt he had become morose and withdrawn. . . . During a period when his family was gone for six hours, he ingested an unknown quantity of diazepam. In the ICU he expressed his wish to die with dignity should complications develop, stressing the meaninglessness of his life as his disability progressed. Examination revealed severe neurological deficits, but no worse than in recent examinations. Psychiatric consultation revealed that the onset of withdrawal and depression coincided with a diagnosis of inoperable cancer in his mother-in-law, with whom his wife was spending more and more time. On the night of the suicide attempt the patient's wife and two sons had left him alone for the first time to visit his mother-in-law.[20]

In Case 1 we would *not* predict that the patient would come to welcome a blood transfusion. Jehovah's Witnesses wish to live, "but not with blood transfusions,"[21] because they believe that a blood transfusion would deprive them of eternal salvation. Hence, criterion (B) is not satisfied, a blood transfusion would be wrong on our criteria, and this is consistent with our considered moral judgment that Jehovah's Witnesses should not be compelled to receive blood transfusions for which they have not consented. In Case 2, however, the paternalistic intervention is justified because we expect that the patient would come to welcome life-prolonging interventions that may be necessary, at least once he was helped to communicate his needs to his family. That, in fact, was the outcome: "The patient had too much pride to complain to his wife about his feelings of abandonment. . . . Discussion with all four family members lead to improved communication and acknowledgment of the patient's special emotional needs. After these conversations, the patient explicitly retracted both his suicidal threats and his demand that no supportive medical efforts be undertaken."[22] Applying our criteria in both cases justifies precisely what we take to be the proper course of action in each. These cases provide additional support for our confidence in the soundness of using criteria (A), (B) and (C) to justify or condemn paternalistic interventions.

THE PRACTICAL IMPLICATIONS
OF THESE RESULTS

Our results to this point show that if we are to continue treating patients against their expressed wishes in cases of serious bodily injury, we must begin an investigation to insure that what we are doing is justified. Our current practices must be measured against the evidence already available, viz., whatever follow-up reports there are on patients who have been kept alive against their wishes. Every suicide by a former burn victim or cervical spinal cord victim who wished to be allowed to die raises nagging doubts about whether keeping the person alive was the right course of action, whereas every interview in which the patient is grateful is some evidence for continuing such interventions. Our current care of such patients need not change as long as there is no reasonable suspicion that we are keeping alive badly injured patients who would later only resent our interference. But follow-up work on such patients has not been thoroughly carried out.[23] To fail to begin such research into the attitudes of those we have kept alive against their wishes is to continue to rely on convenient conventions or on "hunches," and so to be willing to take the chance that what we are doing is morally wrong.

The aim of the research for which I am calling is to gain evidence that will permit us to identify those badly injured patients who are likely to welcome the medical treatments that they are currently refusing. The beginning format of such research involves interviewing patients who have been severely burned or have suffered cervical spinal cord injury to see what they think about the value of their lives and the worth of the intervention. A number of questions would need to be answered, and the following list is not intended to be exhaustive:

1. After your injury, did you consent to the medical treatments that were required to keep you alive?
2. Do you recall whether your explicit consent to or your rejection of life-saving treatment was an inner and settled conviction, or did you feel unsure?
3. If you now contracted a blood infection that could be rather easily cured but otherwise would cause you to become unconscious and to die painlessly in a matter of days, would you consent to be treated for the infection?
4. If you could return to the time of your injury and and have the medical staff do precisely what you wished, in light of what you now know, would you ask to be treated for your injury or only to be treated for your pain?
5. If another person much like yourself suffered an injury as you did, and the medical staff asked your opinion on what the staff should do, what would you say?

These questions may seem psychologically distressful to ex-patients, but persons who have undergone such traumas are typically much more comfortable with these and other troublesome topics — sex, work, loneliness — than are most of us who project our own insecurities into their situations. There is, of course, nothing sacrosanct about the form of the above questions, but what must be discovered is:

Was this a patient who was able to express consent? Was consent expressed?
What was the patient's inner conviction at the time, if any?
Does the patient now generally find life worth living?
Does the patient generally think that the intervention was worthwhile?
Does he or she generally welcome it?

The answers to these questions will likely vary with the kind of injury (e.g., burn or spinal cord), the severity of the injury, the time elapsed since the injury, the time elapsed since the patient no longer needed acute medical treatment, the age of the patient, the patient's sex, the patient's race, the social supports available to the person, the person's economic status, whether or not the person has a suicidal history, whether or not the person has a drug or alcohol history, whether or not the person feels responsible for the injury, whether or not any other persons were hurt or killed, and so on. The list of potential relevant factors will be extensive, and one of the challenges of the research will be to try to identify social, personal, medical, and other factors that may allow us to isolate relevant differences among patients. Depending on the answers patients give to the questions that must be asked, further puzzles and new dead ends may be created, but there will also be some headway as well as a greater appreciation of what we in fact do in keeping such patients alive against their wishes.

This research, ideally, will lead to one of three results. (1) We may discover, for some identifiable group of patients who refused treatment, that most of these patients came to welcome the intervention that they formerly refused. If these are our findings, we have justified the practice of keeping these patients alive against their wishes, and, of course, we should continue the practice of doing so. (2) We may, however, discover that some groups of patients tend to commit suicide shortly thereafter, or tend not to maintain life-prolonging therapies, or, *what is equally definitive from an ethical point of view*, condemn the medical profession for having prevented them from dying earlier. If we do uncover such widespread rejection by a group of patients, then, because we are not ethically justified in keeping alive a patient who will not likely come to welcome our intervention, we have no realistic option but to stop keeping badly injured persons in this group alive against their wishes.[24] (3) We may also discover that the few survivors of some severe injuries, most of whom we allowed to die out of compassion, welcome the treatment they previously tried to reject. If these are our findings, we have grounds for extending paternalistic treatment to all similar cases.

The results of this research are likely to be of help to medical personnel who care for badly injured patients who want to die. Some bioethicists have argued, for instance, that we should let such patients die.[25] The providers of such care clearly do not agree and they frequently keep such patients alive.[26] The bioethicists in question, in their defense of liberty, accuse the medical providers of violating the rights of patients, whereas the medical practitioners see bioethicists as outsiders who are making a very difficult job even harder. (The difficulty of the job is typified by the remark of one nurse who works with burn victims: "Twenty-four hours a day we inflict pain."[27]) In many cases, I believe, the research I am calling for will justify the medical practitioner and provide justificatory protection and even solace to persons working in some of the most difficult areas of patient care.

Whatever we discover, the results are likely to generate a complexity and controversy that will require further conceptual work after the preliminary research is well underway. For example, suppose that a patient comes to welcome the intervention only after many years. Does this show we were right in intervening, or only that this patient has forgotten how painful the treatments, grief, and life-changes were? Or, to take a different problem, suppose 50 or 60 percent of the patients come to welcome (or reject) the interventions, rather than 80 or 90 percent? And suppose there seem to be no further relevant distinctions or categorizations we can employ that will allow us to segregate those who come to welcome (or reject) interventions from those who do not? Although we could speculate about these and other possible findings, such speculation at this point would only be a distracting form of mental gymnastics. Our findings, of themselves, will provide not only some important answers, but also new controversies.

A general objection to this approach that has been raised by some bioethicists is worth discussing before I close. Some persons may be uncomfortable treating patients against their will if one out of ten will not come to welcome the treatment, and others may be uncomfortable in failing to treat if only one out of ten will come to welcome the life-saving treatments.[28] Such discomfort, however, does not reflect the status of our moral obligations in a world in which everything is uncertain, including the outcomes of most medical protocols. If we apply the Kantian ethic and try to do our best to respect the deeper will of a person under severe duress, then we do that by intervening if the odds are very high—say nine out of ten—that we are doing what the person will welcome after the period of stress has passed. On the other hand, we fail to respect the person's autonomy if the odds are very high that the person will not come to welcome our intervention, yet we intervene anyway. So, too, acting on good but inconclusive evidence is justified on a utilitarian ethic.[29] If the odds are very high that the person will assess that the suffering is offset by the positive quality of his or her life, then we are doing what will likely bring about the best results if we treat similar recalcitrant patients. If the odds are very high that the person will not think the treatments are made worthwhile by the subsequent quality of life, then to treat such a person is to do what will likely bring about unnecessary suffering. For anyone who still feels that we cannot act morally unless we are absolutely certain of the results, it must be pointed out that everything we do in life we do under conditions of uncertainty. The following remarks from the opening passages of Aristotle's *Nicomachean Ethics* are relevant: "Our discussion will be adequate if it achieves clarity within the limits of the subject matter. For precision cannot be expected in the treatment of all subjects alike, any more than it can be expected in all manufactured articles. . . . A well-schooled person is one who searches for that degree of precision in each kind of study which the nature of the subject at hand admits."[30] This is the general procedure we follow in medicine and elsewhere in our lives, and not to follow it in ethics would be debilitatingly irrational.

Our conclusions point to an important kind of research that must begin if we are to make headway in justifying, on some objective grounds, daily medical interventions and their omissions in cases involving burn victims and cervical spinal cord injury patients. This research, in turn, must be interdisciplinary in nature, for it requires the ability to bring into play the key conceptual and ethical points discussed above, the insight and experience to identify those features that might allow us to distinguish among relevant categories of patients, and the skill to conduct the required interviews with openness and compassion. The results of such research will, most likely, raise new questions as much as they resolve old ones. But to fail to proceed with such an investigation is to be unresponsive to the relevant conceptual and ethical considerations and, as a result, to take the chance of making life and death decisions on the basis of values and intuitions that may have little to do with the values and character of the patients in question. I hope that this essay will serve as a catalyst for the serious work of finding out just what burn victims, quadraplegics, and others whom we have kept alive against their wishes think we have done to them, for the results of this research will put to rest many of those ethical controversies that make caring for these patients more difficult than it has to be.[31]

NOTES TO CHAPTER 11

1. Some writers distinguish between violations of liberty and restrictions of freedom. See, for example, Bernard Gert and Charles M. Culver, "Paternalistic Behavior," *Philosophy and Public Affairs* 6, no. 1 (1976): 45–57, especially note 4.

2. For example, see Gordon Harper, "The Burn Unit," in Thomas Hackett and Ned Cassem, eds., *Massachusetts General Hospital Handbook of General Hospital Psychiatry* (Saint Louis: The C.V. Mosby Company, 1978), especially pp. 407–413.

3. In this rough definition of paternalism, I follow Gert and Culver, "Paternalistic Behavior," although for another influential definition, see Gerald Dworkin, "Paternalism," *The Monist* 56, no. 1 (June, 1972): 64–84.

4. No one insists upon aggressive treatment in cases in which survival is unprecedented, although such patients may be offered a full therapeutic regimen if they would like. See Sharon Imbus and Bruce Zawacki, "Autonomy for Burned Patients When Survival is Unprecedented," *New England Journal of Medicine* 297, no. 6 (1975): 308–311.

5. Bruce Miller, "Autonomy and Refusing Lifesaving Treatment," *The Hastings Center Report* 11, no. 4 (August 1981), p. 27.

6. H. Tristram Engelhardt, "A Demand to Die," *The Hastings Center Report* 4 (1975), p. 11.

7. Arthur Dyck, "An Alternative to the Ethics of Euthanasia," in Reiser, et al., eds., *Ethics in Medicine* (Cambridge, Mass.: MIT Press, 1977), p. 533.

8. Kant, *Foundations of the Metaphysics of Morals* (Indianapolis, Indiana: The Bobbs-Merrill Company, Inc., 1959): 47.

9. Robert Nozick, *Anarchy, State, and Utopia* (New York: Basic Books, Inc., 1974), p. 31.

10. For a relevant distinction between choices and unrealistic wishes, see Aristotle, *Nicomachean Ethics*, 1111b–1112a.

11. Richard Brandt offers a very thorough discussion of how depression alters rational assessment in "The Morality and Rationality of Suicide," in James Rachels, ed., *Moral Problems* (New York: Harper & Row, 1971): 363–387.

12. On utilitarian grounds, the rightness or wrongness of an act does not depend on what *actually* happens, but on what was *likely* to happen *given the evidence available to the agents at the time of action*. For more on

the interpretation of utilitarianism, see B. Gruzalski, "Forseeable Consequence Utilitarianism," *Australasian Journal of Philosophy* 59 (June
1981): 163–176.

13. John Stuart Mill, *Utilitarianism* (Indianapolis, Indiana: The Bobbs–Merrill
Company, Inc., 1975), p. 10.

14. L.H. Roth, et al., in "Tests of Competency to Consent to Treatment,"
American Journal of Psychiatry 134 (1977): 279–284, point out that
competency is rarely determined as an independent variable.

15. There may, of course, be other evidence that in specific cases will seem
more important than what the ex-patient reports. For example, it might be
that the patient is deceiving himself about the quality of his life but refuses to admit that deception to himself because it would be too painful
psychologically. Or it might be that the patient believes that he ought to
have died (perhaps he was given a blood transfusion against his religious
convictions) and cannot psychologically admit that his life is so good that
it justifies the suffering he went through in order to stay alive. Although
in such cases the observations of others might be better evidence than the
explicit report of the ex-patient about the ex-patient's assessment of
whether the intervention was worth it, to rely on such third party reports
would be to overlook the fact that third parties themselves have vested
interests that may prevent them from correctly assessing what is worthwhile to the ex-patient. Hence, it seems that we must, at least at the start,
focus on ex-patient reports as the most reliable evidence available.

16. Matt Clark, et al., "When Doctors Play God," *Newsweek*, 31 August 1981,
p. 53.

17. The problem illustrated by this example is discussed by, among others,
Rosemary Carter in "Justifying Paternalism," *Canadian Journal of Philosophy* 7 (1977): 133–145.

18. Contrast this with Rosemary Carter's criterion, *Ibid.*, p. 138, viz.: that
it not be true that the act in question is casually sufficient for the subsequent consent.

19. This first case is based on the discussion of cases of Jehovah's Witnesses in
Samuel Gorovitz, et al., eds., *Moral Problems in Medicine* (Englewood
Cliffs, New Jersey: Prentice-Hall, Inc., 1976), pp. 234–241.

20. David L. Jackson and Stuart Youngner, "Patient Autonomy and 'Death
with Dignity,'" *The New England Journal of Medicine* 301 (1979), p. 406.

21. Bruce Miller, "Autonomy," p. 22.

22. Jackson and Younger, "Patient Autonomy," p. 406.

23. Although there has been a lot of follow-up with children, very little has
been done with adults, and what has been done does not focus on what
they would now wish had been done to them. For a recent study, see
N.J.C. Andreasen, et al., "Psychiatric Complications in the Severely
Burned," *Annals of Surgery* 174 (November 1971): 785–793.

24. A logical alternative would be to so improve the quality of these persons' lives that they now think that their paternalistic treatments have been made worthwhile, but this option is a pipedream, especially given the current political climate.

25. For example, Engelhardt, "A Demand to Die," pp. 9–11.

26. "Caring for the Burned," *Life* 3, no. 3 (March 1980).

27. *Ibid.*, p. 119.

28. Donald Van De Veer, "Paternalism and Subsequent Consent," *Canadian Journal of Philosophy* IX, no. 4 (December 1979), p. 640.

29. See Supra, note 12.

30. Aristotle, *Nicomachean Ethics*, 1094b 10–25.

31. I am indebted to comments and suggestions made by William DeAngelis, Carl Nelson, Stephen Nathanson, Sharon B. Young, and the members of the first year medical school class to whom I presented this material in the spring of 1981 at Tufts Medical School.

12 TECHNOLOGY ASSESSMENT IN MEDICAL CARE
Appraisal and Conflict Resolution

Seymour Perry

The technology of medicine, that is, the application of scientific development to clinical care, is becoming increasingly complex and costly. Moreover, although many technological advances replace older, less effective ones, many do not; they are true advances, the first incursion against heretofore untreatable situations. Medical technology combined with the onrush of fundamental biomedical discoveries is constantly changing the face of medicine. The quality of medical care in this country has been rising for over a hundred years, and we seem to be on the brink of a new wave of developments that may make current practice seem as obsolete tomorrow as we consider leeching today.

Yet not all new developments are useful. Not all are sufficient advances over current technologies to warrant their extra cost. There are technologies that have unexpected economic, ethical, and social side effects. Gastric freezing of ulcers, for example, was not a successful innovation. There are many ophthalmologists who question the value of intraocular lens implants compared to routine cataract surgery. Therapeutic abortion is still the focus of ongoing debate in this country. The introduction of continuous-flow analyzers may drop the per-test cost for laboratory procedures, but encourage the ordering of many unnecessary tests as part of a package, at an increase in actual costs.

It is clear that technological innovation is not value-free, and that sometimes the costs are not only economic, but otherwise unforseeable. Gardner Dozois, the science fiction writer, recently wrote that from knowledge of the automobile and the motion picture, the drive-in movie could have been extrapolated. What was unforseeable was the effect of the drive-in on the sexual behavior of American teenagers.

There is increasing emphasis on the evaluation of technological innovation for three major reasons, then:

- Questions of efficacy, which concern themselves with the quality of health care;

- Questions of economics, focusing on costs to the individual and to society; and

- Questions of social policy and ethics.

MEDICAL TECHNOLOGY APPRAISAL IN OTHER COUNTRIES

The United States is not alone in its recognition of the need for the assessment of biomedical technologies. Most advanced industrial nations support, at least to some extent, medical technology assessments of one sort or another.

In Great Britain, with its well-known medical care system, clinical performance and clinical trials are the major facets of evaluation. There is, however, little attention paid to evaluating the social or economic impacts of innovation. The Department of Health and Social Security and the Social Service Research Council may support some studies, and some work on evaluating the impact of technologies may be done independently in universities.

The evaluation of medical technologies in Japan is founded on peer and professional endorsement following introduction by eminent clinicians. This process applies to all forms of technology—drugs, devices, and procedures. Once a technology has been replicated and modified, it is introduced to the Pharmaceutical Affairs Bureau of the Ministry of Health and Welfare for review and approval.

The general evaluation of new biomedical technologies in Sweden is performed by selected physicians, prominent in their specialties, who are consultants to the National Board of Health and Welfare. They essentially assess the efficacy of the technology in question. If the technology seems likely to fulfill unmet medical needs, another governmental body formulates a plan to make the technology more widely available.

In West Germany efficacy studies, such as clinical trials, and cost-effectiveness studies are rare. In part this is due to a shortage of analytically trained statisticians, epidemiologists, health operations researchers, and health planners. However, the government has ear-marked substantial resources for training the necessary professionals. This is an example of West Germany's growing awareness of the need for review of the safety and efficacy of new technologies.

Medical procedures in France are not subject to any governmental evaluation. Drugs, however, must meet standards of safety and efficacy to be sold in France, and these decisions are made with the assistance of expert commissions. Although medical devices are not evaluated for efficacy before being marketed, the national sickness insurance fund may provide limited reimbursement for a new device in return for assistance in evaluating efficacy, an effort undertaken by either a government or a university group.

Although most countries have done little to assure the timely evaluation of medical technologies, the need for such evaluation has become evident to most. Furthermore, a number of countries, such as France, West Germany, and the Netherlands, are attempting to expand their evaluative efforts.

MEDICAL TECHNOLOGY ASSESSMENT IN THE UNITED STATES

In the United States, responsibility for governmental assessment of health care technologies has been located in the Department of Health and Human Services (HHS). Within the Department, assessments of technologies pertinent to health care occur on two levels. The National Institutes of Health (NIH), representing interest and expertise in the biomedical sciences, has emphasized technical consensus development—the assessment of scientific and medical aspects of the technology in question. Other agencies in this department also engage in evaluation activities on a smaller scale. The recently established National Center for Health Care Technology is responsible for coordinating all the assessment activities in the Department, and has a mandate for assessing economic, social, legal, and ethical implications of technologies along with scientific and medical issues.

In this chapter, I will discuss in some depth the two types of assessment activities: (1) those dealing with purely medical aspects and (2) those concerned with social implications.

CONSENSUS DEVELOPMENT PROGRAM OF THE NIH

The primary goal of the consensus development program of the NIH is to improve the translation of the results of biomedical research into knowledge that can be used effectively in the practice of medicine. Its specific responsibilities are to facilitate and coordinate technical consensus-development activities at the NIH, to improve the translation of the results of medical research pertinent to health care into information useful to the practicing community, and to monitor the progress and effectiveness of NIH technology assessment activities.

The consensus development program is a new development, but in the range of assessment activities, clinical trials are prominent. NIH supports many such trials at a cost of millions of dollars. This country has been and continues to be the leader for both terms of trials and their quality. Of course, our stringent drug approval requirements as administered by the Food and Drug Administration (FDA) is in part the driving force for these trials.

The consensus development program, the principal NIH-wide approach to the assessment of health care technologies, consists of activities that bring together various concerned parties to seek general agreement on the safety, efficacy, and appropriate conditions for use of various medical procedures, drugs, and devices. The NIH acts as a catalyst, providing the initiative and the resources to allow appropriate members of the medical professions, the research community, consumers, and others to join in evaluating a technology.

On the basis of experience to date, the consensus development mechanism fosters the production of recommendations that are likely to receive wide acceptance. Its aim is to identify both the valid advances and the gaps in a given field of knowledge, using the experience and expertise of various individuals and organizations to ensure an ample, balanced foundation for conclusions. The opportunity for open discussion and public debate helps to clarify findings, issues, and points of view. Active participation of all concerned parties in the decisionmaking process promotes the acceptance and application of the conclusions reached.

In the assessment of health care technologies, the consensus development program has held conferences at the culmination of the evaluation process. Such conferences serve a different purpose from traditional state-of-the-art conferences, which address the status of research on a particular topic with limited discussion among persons with diverse viewpoints. Consensus development conferences, on the other hand, focus on the application or potential application in health care delivery.

Consensus development activities also differ from the science-court approach in which managers, acting as lawyers, present scientific fact to be adjudicated by neutral judges versed in that particular science. Judgment in a science court is based only on scientific fact, separated from social, moral, economic, or political implications. Unlike consensus development, such proceedings involve only invited participants; the outcome may not reflect a broad consensus.

It is important to ensure that the conference aimed at seeking consensus is open and broadly representative and that audience participation is encouraged. All consensus development conferences are free and open to the public; announcements are widely published and distributed. Biomedical scientists, clinicians, and others in the audience have made important contributions to consensus development, and statements by health care consumers have influenced the outcomes of several conferences, notably those on antenatal diagnosis, intraocular lens implantation, the management of breast cancer, and estrogen use in postmenopausal women. Consensus development panels have been carefully constituted to reflect the range of individuals and organizations with expertise and interest in the use of the technologies; they have included researchers in relevant fields, members of the pertinent clinical specialties, health care consumers, and others. When appropriate, representatives of consumer advocate groups and the general public have also been included. Care has been taken to include women and members of minority groups. In most instances, conference planners have chosen to use neutral panels, whose members do not have publicly stated opinions on the issues being addressed, but some of the panels have been adversary in nature, representing, in so far as possible, a balance of opposing viewpoints.

At times, consensus—defined in this context as general agreement among all or nearly all the panelists—has not been obtained on the answers to one or more questions. The inability to reach a consensus on such matters as efficacy and safety usually indicates that the knowledge base is inadequate. Those preparing consensus statements have been instructed to note those areas in which conclusions cannot yet be reached and to identify the areas in which further research is needed. When one or a very few participants have disagreed with the accepted recommendations, they have been encouraged to submit minority reports stating their views.

Initially, there was some concern over the reception that the medical community might give the consensus development program. Some were apprehensive that clinicians would misconstrue consensus development as a federal attempt to dictate the practice of medicine rather than an attempt to synthesize the best current opinions to assist the profession in clinical decisionmaking. However,the general reaction to date has been highly positive, both in the practicing community and among the specialties.

Concern also existed that consensus development would tend to stifle innovation. However, considerable care has been taken to present consensus statements not as pronouncements, but as conclusons that can be soundly drawn from available information. Indeed, the emphasis on the inclusion of recommendations for further research actually fosters innovation and has helped policymakers to identify areas of opportunity. Recognizing that changes in technology, availability of new data, and other factors can render previous conclusions obsolete, there is an effort underway to develop a process to update consensus sta tements on a continuing basis.

ASSESSMENT ACTIVITIES OF THE NATIONAL CENTER FOR HEALTH CARE TECHNOLOGY

The National Center for Health Care Technology was established by law in 1978 when Congress identified the need in the executive branch for a formal entity with a mandate to evaluate technologies in health care. The Center's assessments fall into two main categories:

1. Multifaceted assessments of technologies identified by the Center, The National Council on Health Care Technology, the Assistant Secretary for Health, and others as being of high priority. By means of the assessment process, information is synthesized, separating out the pertinent issues and identifying those areas which require further research, demonstrations, or evaluation; and

2. Research, demonstrations, and evaluations addressing specific aspects of technologies (i.e., safety, efficacy, effectiveness, and their cost-effectiveness, and social, ethical, and economic impacts).

Although each technology presents a unique set of considerations and thus requires an individualized approach, the Center has adopted certain principles in structuring its assessments. In particular, the Center emphasizes three specific goals:

1. To utilize processes that foster valid and reproducible assessments of health care technologies. To this end the Center attempts to support the development and application of reliable methodologies in data gathering and analysis.

2. To provide a means for individuals and organizations, both within and outside the government, to gather information, perform research and assessments, or develop recommendations. Whenever appropriate, the Center cosponsors or complements technology assessments conducted by other organizations or agencies, and encourages broad participation so that all individuals with significant information and viewpoints have the opportunity to contribute.

3. To promote the broad and timely dissemination of findings through its own publications, scientific and medical journals, the National Library of Medicine, and other channels. Thus, the Center uses existing modalities for information dissemination while developing additional innovative approaches to distribute this information in its most useful form to its consumers. The target audiences include the health professions, the public, federal agen-

cies with responsibilities in health and health care reimbursement, and the health care industry.[1]

Multifaceted assessments are integrated analyses of the safety, efficacy, effectiveness, and social, ethical, and economic issues of technology. Largely on the basis of recommendations from the Council, the Secretary of HHS, the Assistant Secretary for Health, the Department's Technology Coordinating Committee (TCC), and others, the Center identifies technologies for these extensive evaluations. They may range from emerging and new technologies to established preventive, diagnostic, therapeutic, and rehabilitative technologies. The criteria for identifying priority technologies include:

1. The actual or potential risks and the actual or potential benefits to patients associated with the use of the technology;
2. The actual or potential cost of the technology;
3. The actual or potential rate of its use; and
4. The stage of development of the technology.[2]

These criteria, which the Council has further refined, indicate that a preliminary review of an identified technology is necessary to ascertain the key issues posed to determine the factors that make the technology of high priority for assessment.

Although the specific format varies with the topic, the usual sequence includes:

*   Commissioning an overview paper
*   Establishing a federal planning group
*   Establishing a full nonfederal planning group
*   Commissioning studies under grant or contract, designed to address the key issues surrounding the technology in question
*   Convening conference(s)

When issues are clarified either through the multifaceted assessment process or otherwise (e.g., a research grant), the Center supports assessments of technologies from one perspective or another through its extramural and intramural programs. Research designed to provide information in areas upon which national policy decisions will be based receives priority. The scientific and technical merit of the research must be demonstrated to peer review groups prior to funding and implementation.

Throughout the assessment process, the Center acts mainly as a catalyst, bringing together those throughout society who have relevant interests, experience, information, and expertise, thus fostering the formulation of valid and reliable findings. In order to minimize bias, the Center ensures that practicing physicians, clinicians in the research community, other investigators from a wide range of biomedical and behavioral disciplines, representatives of the health industry, economists, ethicists, lawyers, members of the general public, and others participate actively in its assessment process at appropriate stages. Often, other Public Health Service (PHS) agencies and agencies outside HHS may assume major roles in the assessments (e.g., The National Institutes of Health (NIH), Food and Drug Administration (FDA), and The Center for Disease Control (CDC) provide medical and scientific evaluations of many of the technologies under assessment).

Earlier, I discussed the NIH consensus development program and noted that it focuses on medical aspects of technologies. When the interests of the Center happen to coincide with that of the NIH, the evaluation is jointly planned. In any case, in mounting an assessment effort the Center seeks the involvement of all the federal agencies that have a programmatic interest in the technology under consideration, including the NIH.

Thus far the Center working with NIH has sponsored evaluations of the Papanicolaow smear, endoscopy in upper gastrointestinal hemorrhage, and birth by cesarian delivery. In December 1980 it joined with the National Heart, Lung, and Blood Institute (NHLBI) in evaluating the medical aspects of coronary artery bypass surgery— the economic, ethical, and other issues were addressed at a conference in April 1981.[3] Evaluations and planning activities are well along for dental X rays and the management of end-stage renal disease, including dialysis and transplantation. Planning has been initiated for a number of other technologies, including hip replacement, cerebral artery bypass surgery, and screening for neural tube defects.

The Center has also provided Medicare with recommendations on forty-five technologies about which there were reimbursement questions. The creation of the Center strengthened the linkage between Health Care Financing Administration (HCFA) and The Public Health Service, which required Medicare to turn to the Center for advice in setting coverage policies.[4]

OPPOSITION TO THE CENTER

Despite the obvious benefits of assessment activities, there has been criticism of assessment programs by at least two groups—the American Medical Association (AMA) and the Health Industry Manufacturers Association (HIMA). This and other opposition gained momentum in the antiregulatory mood of the Reagan administration and the 1981–82 Congress.

The AMA's strong opinion on reauthorization of the Center is based in particular upon statutory language that authorizes the evaluation of modes and techniques of *all* phases of medical practice. Believing that "relevant clinical policy analysis and judgments are better made, and are being responsibly made, within the medical profession," the AMA has forcefully argued against the Center.

> A centralized government authority, a National Center for Health Care Technology, created to orchestrate medical technology assessment, diffusion, and use—as well as ethical judgments and social decisions—cannot and should not supplant the current diverse system. This is especially so when the mandate of such authority is essentially to facilitate the achievement of economic, not health goals, to make definitive reimbursement recommendations that cannot begin fairly to reflect the complex and changing circumstances that a physician, patient and a local community must deal with.[5]

The Health Industry Manufacturers Association's principle concern continues to be with the potential stifling of innovation they fear a technology assessment program may induce. They have argued that assessments should not focus on emerging medical technologies until promising technologies are "exposed to the rigors of clinical settings to demonstrate both (their) merits and shortcomings."

> Assessments of safety, effectiveness, cost-effectiveness, social acceptability, and other aspects of any medical technology are developed over time by the interaction of firms and individuals in a market environment. Producers must demonstrate the features of their products and in many instances must make modifications to satisfy the needs of consumers. Otherwise, markets for the items collapse.[6]

I believe that the actual performance of the Center since its inception in 1978 effectively answers these critics. The NIH consensus conferences have drawn the most recognizably knowledgable physicians and researchers together to insure comprehensive and diverse discussion and analysis. These forums have sought to influence clinical practice with the best and most up-to-date judgments on procedures and treatments that only the experts can be really knowledgable about. The evaluation of modern medicine simply requires more rigor than is commonly afforded in an ad hoc and imperfect marketplace. And in so far as the Center's recommendations influence reimbursement policies, its goal is making sure that only *beneficial* therapies are paid for. Recently, the Center for Analyses of Health Practices at the Harvard School of Public Health estimated that four specific recommendations of the National Center for Health Care Technology not to reimburse because of unproved effectiveness would lead to a savings of $312 million to Medicare and $1 billion to the public over a 10-year period.

The vigorous opposition to the Center by the AMA and HIMA and by supporters of the administration, particularly in the senate, led to a struggle in the Congress between those who wanted to see it abolished and those who favored its continuation. Mainly due to the commitment and leadership of Congressman Waxman, Democrat of California, the Center was reauthorized for three years when the Budget Reconciliation Act of 1981 was passed in the summer of that year. During the deliberations, a large number of organizations spoke out in support of the Center, including the American College of Physicians, the Association of American Medical Colleges, major third party payers, and the Association for the Advancement of Medical Instrumentation. Nevertheless, the administration and the Office of Management and Budget, presumably at the urging of the AMA and HIMA, refused to alter their opposition to the Center. The administration's position prevailed in the Congress and no funds were provided for the Center when the appropriations bills were passed in late 1981. The Center effectively ceased to exist in December, 1981, so that at the present time in the government there is no formal medical technology assessment program of the scope provided by the Center.

CONCLUSION

The assessment of biomedical technologies is an expanding effort worldwide. Here in the United States, biomedical technology assessments are supported to a greater degree and a broader scope than in any other developed country. When one considers that the most significant efforts to assess biomedical technologies in Europe are made in those countries where the government manages the provision of health services, the depth and extent of the American effort is all the more remarkable, for here there is no infringement on the practice of medicine, nor is there limitation of innovation through technology assessment. This flexibility is a result of the creative partnership of government, industry, and professional societies all working together to develop the best possible information about particular technologies.

The establishment of the National Center for Health Care Technology introduced a new factor into the biomedical research/health care delivery system—one that I believe was overdue and essential in our society. The failure of the Congress to appropriate funds for the continued operation of the Center deprives health policymakers, third party payers, the medical profession, and others of a valuable source of information concerning medical technologies, their safety, efficacy, and societal implications. Technological innovation has brought us enormous advances as well as hitherto unknown problems and complexities. An entity such as the Center is essential if we are to address these problems intelligently and responsibly.

NOTES TO CHAPTER 12

1. Seymour Perry and John T. Kalberer, "The NIH Consensus-Development Program and the Assessment of Health-Care Technologies," *The New England Journal of Medicine* 303 (1980): 169–172.
2. Section 309 of the Public Health Service Act (The Health Services Research, Health Statistics and Health Care Technology Act of 1978): P.L. 95–623; and "Procedures, Priorities and Policy for Assessment of Health Care Technology." National Center for Health Care Technology, Dept. of Health and Human Services, 1981.
3. "Report from the NCHCT: Coronary Artery Bypass Surgery." NCHCT Technology Assessment Forum. *J.A.M.A.* 246 (1981): 1645–1649.
4. Public Health Service Medical and Scientific Evaluation of Health Care Technologies. Assessment Report Series Vol. 1 (Department of Health and Human Services, 1981).
5. Joseph F. Boyle, M.D., "Statement of the American Medical Association," (Subcommittee on Health and the Environment, Committee on Energy and Commerce, U.S. House of Representatives) March 20, 1981: 6.
6. Robert A. Schoellhorn, "Testimony of the Health Industry Manufacturers Association," (Subcommittee on Health and the Environment, Committee on Energy and Commerce, U.S. House of Representatives) March 20, 1981: 2.

13 AN AGENDA FOR MEDICAL ETHICS

Samuel Gorovitz

In the last decade, medical ethics has emerged as an identifiable and highly visible field of inquiry. There is much interest in it on the part of scholars in many disciplines, health care providers, students, representatives of the news media, and the public. At the same time, there is deep dissatisfaction with it in many quarters. I believe the dissatisfaction is justified in an important way, and that the time has come for the discipline to undergo a corrective change in direction. My purpose here is to state the case and describe the change that I see as needed.

HISTORICAL BACKGROUND

Although concern with the moral aspects of medical care is ancient, such issues were historically addressed primarily within the medical profession and by those who sought, through legislative action, to protect or advance the public interest by the advocacy of legal con-

I am grateful to the National Center for Health Services Research, with whom I worked during the time that the ideas expressed here took form. I am also grateful for helpful conversations with the staffs of the Hastings Center, the Kennedy Center for Bioethics, and the Health Policy Program of the University of California at San Francisco, and with numerous others at Stanford, the Pacific School of Religion, the California Department of Health, and several hospitals in San Francisco.

straints or entitlements pertaining to matters of health care. In these areas, and to a lesser extent in a few other related areas, there is a history of published discussion of the moral issues in health care. More recently, those moral issues have aroused dramatically increased professional and public attention because of the dramatically increased efficacy of medical and scientific procedures, their greater visibility through the mass media, the spectacular rise in the costs associated with health care, and changing social expectations with respect to health services.

The agenda of problems that provides the focus for work in medical ethics has gone through three stages thus far. In an earlier era, when considerations of medical ethics took place largely within the medical community, the phrase "medical ethics" would frequently be taken to refer to a variety of issues concerning the conventions of medical practice. That tradition of inquiry was reflected as recently as 1972, when the Judicial Council of the American Medical Association issued a statement on the Principles of Medical Ethics in which it addressed attention to such questions as whether physicians should advertise, collect referral commissions, lecture to groups of chiropractors, and the like. To distinguish such questions about the conventions of clinical practice from questions of more substantial philosophical interest, I have referred to the former as questions of professional etiquette.

More recently, the taxonomy of problems in medical ethics came to be viewed differently. Instead of referring to the old issues of professional etiquette, "medical ethics" was understood to refer to a new variety of problems, characterizable largely in essentially medical or biological terms. Thus, the focus shifted to problems of abortion, birth defects, euthanasia, genetic counseling, experimentation on human subjects, and so on. That taxonomy persists as the most common interpretation of the problems of medical ethics, but it has increasingly been required to share the spotlight with a different taxonomy. Inquiry into many of the medical contexts that generate moral dilemmas reveals certain common threads of philosophical puzzlement. For example, questions about the right to commit suicide, about involuntary confinement, about the Jehovah's Witness's right to refuse blood transfusions, and about whether the adolescent patient should have access to medical treatment in confidence from parents (who perhaps cover its cost) involve issues of personal autonomy and the justifiability of paternalistic intervention.

Similarly, questions about responsibility to sustain the lives of seriously deformed newborn infants, like questions about responsibility to sustain the lives of severely deteriorated, terminally ill victims of injury, illness, or advanced age, raise questions about the value of life and the relevance of considerations of quality of life to the assessment of the value of life. Only a consistent point of view about personal autonomy, the justification of paternalistic intervention, and the considerations that are relevant to determing the value of life in general or a given life in particular can allow one to develop a consistent perspective on the various different problems of medical ethics that are reflected in a medically inspired taxonomy.

There is thus a taxonomy of topics, fundamentally philosophical in conception, that must be addressed as part of the process of dealing with the problems of medical ethics. These philosophical topics are not new, of course. What is new is the extent to which clarity about them has been recognized as necessary for the resolution of problems that arise elsewhere. The topics at issue include: autonomy, coercion, normalcy, naturalness, rights, dependency, justice, responsibility, personhood, and numerous others. As a result, philosophers have become increasingly prominent in the literature of medical ethics, and philosophical concepts appear with frequency even in discussions by others, including physicians who have turned their attention to ethical problems. Still, many observers of the scene have a sense that the issues are not yet properly addressed.

A NEW APPROACH TO MEDICAL ETHICS

There are, I think, two basically different reasons for the dissatisfactions with medical ethics. The first comes under the heading of inappropriate expectations. Some people simply ask too much of medical ethics and the people who pursue it. The discipline can clarify ethical issues and provide insights that can help, to a limited extent, with the resolution of clinical problems or health policy problems that involve moral dilemmas; it cannot, and should not be expected to, provide a way of dissolving such dilemmas simply and painlessly. The question of what it is reasonable to expect of medical ethics is an important one, worth addressing separately.[1] But it is not the issue I want to emphasize here. Rather, I want to focus on the other reason that leads to dissatisfaction with medical ethics.

Because the ethical problems in medicine involve both ethical issues and medical issues, those problems attract attention from philosophically interested physicians and from medically interested philosophers. (Of course, others are involved, too, such as lawyers, theologians, economists, and more; I leave them out not because they are unimportant, but because the point I wish to make can be made more clearly this way.) But all too often the philosophers and the clinical practicioners come to a common problem not only with different backgrounds and viewpoints, but with different objectives as well. The philosopher thus may be attracted to consideration of a problem concerning informed consent because of an interest in the concept of voluntarism, recognizing that the question of when consent is freely given can be a useful question to pursue along the way to a deeper understanding of autonomous action. The physician, on the other hand, may be worried about the same problem of informed consent because of a particularly troublesome, pending case. What counts as success for the philosopher may be an increment of clarity about a general concept; what counts as success for the physician may be help in finding a comfortable approach to the worrisome case; and each may be dissatisfied by what the other finds gratifying. Achieving a meeting of minds is further impeded by the puzzlement that exists outside philosophy about just what the philosopher's methods of research are. Especially to those who come from a tradition of empirical inquiry, the philosopher works in mysterious ways, and hence the credibility of his or her results is often in question. And philosophers typically prefer to remain mute on the subject of their methods, further reinforcing suspicions about the value of what they do. It is time to meet this problem head-on.

In the last five years, there has been a remarkable increase in the literature of medical ethics. Since 1976, at least one new major textbook in the area has appeared each year; there are at least four professional journals under five years old in the area; the number of scholars working as "bioethicists" has increased sharply; the four volume *Encyclopedia of Bioethics* was published in 1978; and increasingly many medical journals are publishing discussions of the ethical problems in clinical practice. There remains, nonetheless, a considerable gap between the discussions in the literature and the problems faced professionally by health service providers and those who have responsibility for the setting and analysis of health policy.

Recent work in medical ethics has tended to focus on problems related to medical research, rather than on individual interactions between provider and patient or on the structural and institutional factors that play a major role in shaping the character of health services in the United States. We spent approximately 5.3 billion dollars on medical research in the fiscal year 1977; that important ethical issues arise in connection with such research is widely recognized, and that recognition was marked by the establishment, by Congress, of the National Commission for the Protection of Human Subjects of Biomedical and Behavioral Research. Since the ethical issues associated with medical research are perennial, even the prodigious accomplishments of that Commission left a long agenda of ethical issues in need of attention. In consequence, in 1979 President Carter appointed the President's Commission for the Study of Ethical Problems in Medicine and Biomedical and Behavioral Research. Although issues in medical practice do fall within the scope of this new Commission, most of the research on ethical issues in medicine that has been done with Federal support thus far has centered on issues that arise in research. Yet health services delivery constitutes a vastly more pervasive factor in contemporary life than does medical research, as evidenced by the fact that in the same fiscal year our expenditure on health care services was approximately 157 billion dollars. And the ethical issues in health care services stand in need of examination at least as much as those in research.

We can redress this imbalance, and at the same time close the gap between the clinician's approach and the philosopher's approach to medical ethics, by embarking on a new agenda of inquiry into ethical problems in health care delivery, conducted as cooperative ventures by those who could reasonably be classified as "bioethicists" working with appropriate colleagues in clinical practice. This will require the development of new methods and new formulations of the questions to be addressed. The sort of research I am suggesting should not address problems of purely theoretical interest, but instead should address ongoing problems in health services delivery or health policy. (This is not to deny or denegrate the value of purely theoretical work; it is simply to call for an additional kind of work.)

The results of the research should be accessible to professionals in broadly divergent disciplines. Such work on the ethics of health services delivery and of health policy should typically include an empirical portion and an analytic portion. The empirical portion would provide an identification and description of the choices made or faced in some area of health services, and of the underlying values that shape such choices. The analytic portion would then provide an assessment of those values in terms of the larger context of broadly shared values—such as respect for liberty, equality, and efficiency— and also in terms of the more idiosyncratic values of individual persons. Research that concentrates on conceptual issues might include an empirical portion descriptive of the importance to health services or health policy of the concepts in question—such as the concept of health or of entitlement of care—and then an analysis that clarifies that concept. In either case, such research should conclude with an account of the consequences for health services delivery or for health policy that should follow from the ethical or conceptual clarification that has been provided. Work of this kind, I believe, is possible, important, and overdue.

IMPROVED RESEARCH METHODOLOGIES

Since the methods of research that are most fruitful in regard to ethical or conceptual problems are themselves a matter of substantial dispute, it is also important to conduct research that leads to methodological clarification and the improvement of research methods. That means that a variety of different methodologies, including experimental approaches, are in order. The following are examples of possible approaches.

1. A great deal has been written about informed consent in both research projects and clinical intervention. Although there continues to be debate about the effects of consent requirements of various degrees of stringency, the importance of the concept of consent is reflected in the law, in government regulations, and in modifications of clinical practice. Philosophers and religious ethicists have sometimes criticised physicians for being insufficiently conscientious in obtaining informed consent, and physicians have sometimes responded by pointing out how uninformed their critics are about the problems of dealing with patients who exhibit varying degrees of intelligence, background information, medical need, fear, denial, and rationality. Even physicians who agree that informed consent require-

ments are appropriate—in recognition of the autonomy of the patient as an independent agent—may be quite uncertain about how and to what extent such a requirement can be met, given the realities of clinical practice.

This problem might be addressed as follows: A physician and philosopher could collaborate on a project designed to examine the various communicative strategies available to a physician seeking to obtain informed consent. Starting with several actual cases, a playwrite working under their direction could prepare scripts of a variety of alternative interactions that could occur—or could have occurred—in the physician's practice. The philosopher could analyze the various approaches with respect to their ethical adequacy, and the physician could assure that the realities of clinical practice are reflected in a credible way in that analysis. The resulting scripts and commentaries could then be used, initially on a test basis, as teaching materials to help house officers learn what sorts of standards and aspirations are reasonable and appropriate in regard to questions of informed consent. Hospital policy could then be evaluated in terms of such standards. As a by-product of the project, the philosopher might come to have a deeper understanding of the problems of clinical practice, and the house officers might come to have a deeper appreciation of the moral foundations of the requirement that informed consent be obtained. Further, the materials that result could perhaps be developed into video tapes that would have wide acceptance in medical schools or teaching hospitals.

2. Among the most pervasive problems in contemporary society is adhering to democratic processes of decision regarding issues that involve great technological complexity. The debates about research involving recombinatory genetics and about the development of nuclear energy are cases in point. No issue seems more complex, however, than that of the regulation and planning of health care programs and facilities. The Health Systems Agencies (HSA) are intended to constitute a mechanism for public involvement in the making of regional health policy decisions, but it is not clear that the currents of information and influence that swirl about the operation of the HSAs provide for solutions that are always in the public interest. Nor is it clear whether or to what extent the decisions of HSAs reflect the best ethical thinking that could be brought to bear on their concerns. A sociologist and a bioethicist with some background in health planning could arrange a temporary affiliation with an HSA

to examine the extent to which ethical issues are recognized by the HSA, the ways in which they are dealt with, and the possibilities for dealing with them more effectively. At some stage in the project, the bioethicist might join the HSA's deliberations, with the sociologist seeking to determine whether, to what extent, and in what ways such an involvement influences the quality of the decisions of the agency, as judged by explicit and defensible criteria.

3. A research group interested in assessing the processes and criteria which determine whether some therapies are admitted into the armamentarium of contemporary health care while others are excluded might be uncertain about which methodology holds the best prospects of clarifying and evaluating the processes and criteria. The group might then refine the methodologies under consideration, to pursue the project in accordance with the methodology judged to be most promising. The group might fail, however, to identify a single methodology among several possibilities that clearly seems to be best. In that case, the group might conduct the project along parallel tracks in two different ways, with two independent subgroups each adopting a different methodology, so that the resulting project would have the dual objectives of clarification of the specific substantive questions and also illumination of the comparative effectiveness of different methodologies.

INTERDISCIPLINARY
MEDICAL-ETHICAL ISSUES

The sort of question that I believe needs to be addressed must combine the empirical realities of the world of health care and health policy with the analytic interests and skills of nonempirical disciplines, typically within the humanities, but with some reliance also on the social sciences. The following areas of possible research will illustrate.

1. A vast literature, including an extensive array of regulations, now exists concerning the ethical aspects of research in health care. Do the arguments and policies that prevail in regard to research apply to the contexts of health services delivery? To what extent are mixed contexts, such as health service demonstration projects, adequately covered by the considerations that have been developed to protect

human subjects in research? For example, are there subjects other than patients who are at risk in demonstration projects—the health care provider, perhaps—and are their interests adequately reflected in present policies?

2. In many states, laws have been enacted covering such matters as licensure, certification, and other issues affecting health services delivery. It should be possible to identify these laws and provide a collective assessment of them to determine: Are these laws consistent with one another? Are they at odds with prevailing medical judgment? Do they serve the public interest? What ought the laws to be in regard to such matters, and for what reasons?

3. What are the appropriate criteria for assessing the quality of health care services? For example, if one mode of treatment adheres strictly to requirements of informed consent, with heightened patient anxiety and a longer period of recovery, as compared with a more paternalistic mode of treatment, by what criteria can we determine which is the better quality care? Are quantitative measures, such as disability days or even days of life, adequate for the assessment of quality of care, or are qualitative factors of primary importance?

4. In regard to practices that are dangerous to varying degrees, to what extent and for what reasons should Federal agencies provide warnings, and to what extent and for what reasons should they ban, regulate, or control?

5. Neonatal intensive care provides a classic example of the conflict between the aspirations of state-of-the-art medical skills and the concerns of values other than sustaining life in all cases. When the survival prospects of 600 gram infants are extremely low, with treatment costs extremely high, and with nursing and other support staff often convinced that continued treatment imposes prolonged psychological and economic hardship on parents, imposes discomfort on the infant, and imposes increased stress on the staff, how should decisions be made about how long to maintain treatment and how long to support it with government funds?

6. Are there special ethical issues associated with long-term chronic care? For example, should economic factors ever be allowed to enter into decisions about treatment? Do the institutionalized structures through which we care for such patients adequately respect their dignity and personal autonomy, or are those structures

ill-fitting applications of structures designed for the delivery of acute care?

7. Are there limits to the responsibility that public health service facilities bear for chronic repeaters—for example, indigent patients who refuse rehabilitative services and reappear regularly as abusive, aggressive, and uncooperative patients? Is any factor other than medical need relevant to the question of entitlement to care?

8. To what extent, under what conditions, should a patient's refusal of treatment be honored? If a patient refuses surgery, as in the case of a gangrenous limb, what are the hospital's continuing obligations to that patient? Is refusal of vitally necessary treatment itself sufficient evidence of incompetence? What ought health care providers do in the face of patient refusals of various sorts, and for what reasons?

9. In this era of coin-operated blood pressure gauges in airports and home-use early pregnancy tests, what is the appropriate policy to advocate about self-diagnosis that does not involve reliance at any point on trained health care professionals? As we envision the development of home-use tests for blood samples or enzyme screening, should the prospect of increasingly sophisticated mechanized self-diagnosis be welcomed or opposed, and for what reasons?

10. What is the appropriate response to patient noncompliance where the patient does not refuse treatment, but rather seeks to exercise an independent judgment about the process of treatment? Does a patient's justified noncompliance exempt the provider from any responsibilities or liabilities? Under what conditions is noncompliance justified? How is it in fact handled in health care settings, and how should it be handled?

11. When nurses are under orders not to disclose a patient's condition to the patient, the patient explicitly and repeatedly asks direct questions that cannot be answered without disclosing information about the diagnosis, and in the nurse's clinical judgment the withholding of information is detrimental to the well-being of the patient, what recourse does the nurse have, and what recourse should the nurse have, when the physician is either unavailable or unwilling to reconsider the issue? Does the structure of health care service provide adequate remedy for those cases in which a nurse is in conflict between the commitment to the patient's interest and the requirements of the hierarchy of authority in the health care setting?

12. What are the conditions under which conscientious refusal to provide health care service is justifiable and should be accepted without resultant penalty? It is widely accepted, even among the proponents of a liberal abortion policy, that no physician should be required to perform an abortion contrary to the dictates of his or her conscience. Are there other situations in which conscientious refusal to perform should be respected?

13. Under what condition are physicians judged to be impaired, and to what extent is the process of review and response adequately protective of the public interest? Are the traditional categories of alcoholism and drug abuse appropriate paradigms of impairment, or should other categories be considered? For example, if a physician, driven by gambling debts or bad investments to seek a larger income, takes more patients than can be handled with the conscientiousness required for competent care, is the physician not also impaired in a way that warrants some measure of external response? What ought the mechanisms of such response be?

14. In a publicly funded fertility and family planning service, are providers justified in taking considerations of parental suitability into account in deciding whether or not to provide treatment? For example, can a person with a record of child abuse or a current problem of narcotics addiction justifiably be denied medical services requested for the purpose of facilitating reproduction? Does it matter that the source of funding for the clinic is public? What obligations do the providers have to whom, and for what reasons, under such circumstances?

15. What are the ethical issues associated with genetic screening, and how are they best resolved? How should the comparative human costs of false negatives and false positives be allocated, when the result of a false positive may be the abortion of a normal child and the result of a false negative may be the birth of a grossly defective child? Should health insurance pay for routine prenatal diagnosis, regardless of the purpose to which the results of such diagnosis may be put? What are the goals of genetic counseling, and by what measures can it be judged successful or unsuccessful?

16. Training competent health care workers requires enabling students and younger practitioners to develop increasing levels of skill by practicing, under supervision, on patients in a variety of circumstances. In some cases, it is common to allow medical procedures

to be performed on the bodies of recently dead patients—especially in the context of emergency medical services—to promote the refinement of medical skills. What ethical issues arise in connection with this aspect of medical training, and how can they best be resolved? Are the rights and legitimate interests of patients adequately respected and protected under present circumstances? Would new guidelines be helpful, or would they place unnecessary additional constraints on valuable opportunities for developing medical expertise?

17. In the effort to contain health care costs, more careful accounting procedures are linking charges ever more closely to patient services actually received. In the process, a part of the funding base for medical education has been eroded. Justice seems to require that patient fees not be used to subsidize the costs of medical education, at least without the consent of the patients or of third-party payers. But the social costs of inadequate support for medical education may be substantial. How then should medical training be financed, with what relationship between the distribution of costs and benefits?

18. Insurance premiums now reflect certain crude measures of the policy holder's health prospects, based on consideration of such factors as family medical history and the policy holder's life-style. As medical prediction becomes more sophisticated, it may become possible to provide far more reliable measures of risk, perhaps based on chromosomal analysis and other predictive techniques. To what extent should insurability or insurance costs be based on such predictive power? Is the concept of insurance itself undermined as the structure of insurance costs increasingly correlates insurance costs and actual medical expenses? Or should individuals bear the burdens of health care costs in proportion to their likely need? Should it matter if that need is a function of behavior, such as smoking or excessive use of alcohol?

19. The concept of competence plays a major role in decisions about the delivery of health care services. Psychological factors and medical circumstances can alter cognitive functioning in such a way as to cause patients to be judged not competent. Considerations of culture, life-style, or age, however, may sometimes cloud the issue, resulting in a judgment of incompetence that reflects the provider's bias more than the patient's limitations. How are such judgments in

fact made? What impact do they have on the quality of health care delivery? How ought they be made?

20. Elderly patients are sometimes categorized, on the basis of rather scant evidence, as requiring nursing home placement. In some settings, the expression "NHP"—nursing home placement—is even used as a diagnostic category at the time of hospital admission. Yet some gerontologists believe that such patients often have medical problems that could be treated in such a way as to make possible either independent living or living in an alternative setting that is preferable to the nursing home. Are the elderly treated with inadequate care because of their age in this or in other respects? To what extent and in what ways are considerations of age relevant to treatment decisions, and for what reasons?

21. Many patients admitted with hypothermia are victims of poverty, climbing utilities costs, and cold winters. The mortality of hypothermia is high, and the treatment of survivors is typically prolonged and costly. Those who survive, however, may then return to the same impoverished environment that caused their illness in the first place. When poverty is the cause of illness, the problem is not inherently medical, but social. Yet its impact on health services and health costs can be substantial. To what extent and in what ways should health care planners attempt to deal with the nonmedical factors that are direct influences on the demand for and cost of health services? When it is clearly less costly to provide a subsidy for the payment of heating bills than to treat hypothermia, should such factors play any role in the scope of planning of health care services provided at public expense or through public agencies?

22. New applications of computer technology to medical contexts prompt increasing concern with related issues of privacy, judgment, and responsibility. Are computerized medical records adequately protected against violation of confidentiality? What is the appropriate definition of 'adequately' in this context? If computerized diagnostic and treatment protocols are developed, can physicians retain the discretion to deviate from such protocols without incurring undue liability?

23. No factor more directly affects the quality of medical care than the character of the person practicing medicine. Many unsuccessful applicants to medical school are intellectually qualified to become physicians, and admission decisions often turn on marginal

considerations. It has been argued that the process selects in a way that is prejudicial to the chances of those applicants who are, in terms of character and motivation, best suited to the practice of clinical medicine. What values are reflected in the way actual medical school admissions decisions are made? Are these the values that it is in the public interest to advance? What revisions in admissions policies, if any, are desirable, and for what reasons?

Each of these areas of inquiry would require the development of an investigative approach that is appropriate to the particular mix of empirical and philosophical issues presented by that area. No general method of inquiry is likely to be suitable for all, or even for many; that may in part account for the notorious inability of the philosopher to give a satisfying account to an inquirer from a scientific field of how philosophers, in general, approach ethical problems in medicine. These projects, nonetheless, could all be pursued to advantage, and it is my conviction that the cumulative weight of such pursuits would be to enhance mutual understanding among the various disciplines that come to bear on the problems of medical ethics, to shrink the gap between the discipline of medical ethics and the concerns about ethics that trouble professionals in health care fields, and to diminish the cloud of dissatisfaction that casts its shadow on the efforts of those who approach the problems of medical ethics from the perspective of any single field.

NOTE TO CHAPTER 13

1.   For an extended discussion of this issue, see S. Gorovitz, *Doctors' Dilemmas: Moral Conflict and Medical Care* (New York: Macmillan, 1982).

INDEX

ABOUT THE CONTRIBUTORS

George J. Annas, J.D., is Associate Professor of Law and Medicine, Boston University School of Medicine, and Chief of the Health Law Section, Boston University School of Public Health. His publications include *Genetics and the Law, Informed Consent to Human Experimentation*, and the two American Civil Liberties Union books, *The Rights of Hospital Patients* and *The Rights of Doctors, Nurses and Allied Health Professionals*.

James L. Bernat, M.D., is chief of Neurology Section, Veterans Administration Hospital, White River Junction, Vermont, and is on the staff of the Division of Neurology of the Department of Medicine, Dartmouth Medical School. He has coauthored several articles on problems in medical ethics that have appeared in such journals as *The Hastings Center Report*.

Christine Cassell, M.D., is an assistant professor in the Department of Medicine and an assistant professor in the Department of Public Health and Preventive Medicine, Oregon Health Sciences University, Portland, Oregon. She is the recepient of the Henry J. Kaiser Family Foundation Faculty Development Award in General Internal Medicine. She has also published a number of articles in medical ethics and has coauthored, with Ruth Purtilo, *Ethical Dimensions in the*

Health Professions. Dr. Cassell is the vice president of Portland Physicians for Social Responsibility.

Charles M. Culver, M.D., Ph.D., is a member of the Department of Psychiatry, Dartmouth Medical School, Hanover, New Hampshire. He has coauthored articles on medical ethics that have appeared in a number of journals, including *The Hastings Center Report* and *Philosophy and Public Policy*, and is the co-author of *Philosophy in Medicine.*

H. Tristram Engelhardt, Jr., M.D., is the Rosemary Kennedy Professor of Medicine at Georgetown University, and Senior Researcher, Kennedy Institute, Center for Bioethics, Georgetown University. He is the author of *Mind–Body: A Categorical Relation*, numerous influencial articles, and a coeditor of the *Encyclopedia of Bioethics*, the *Philosophy and Medicine* series, and, most recently, *Concepts of Health Disease: Interdisciplinary Perspectives.*

Bernard Gert, Ph.D., is Professor of Philosophy at Dartmouth College, Hanover, New Hampshire. He is the author of *The Moral Rules*, editor of Thomas Hobbes's *Man and Citizen*, and co-author of *Philosophy in Medicine*: His articles have appeared in numerous journals, including *Philosophy and Public Affairs* and *The Hastings Center Report.*

Samuel Gorovitz, Ph.D., is professor and Chairman, Department of Philosophy, University of Maryland, College Park, and Senior Scholar, National Center for Health Services Research. His numerous articles have appeared in *The Journal of Philosophy* and elsewhere. He is a coauthor of *Philosophical Analysis: An Introduction to Its Language and Techniques*, the editor of *Freedom and Order in the University*, the senior editor of *Moral Problems in Medicine*, the editor of *Utilitarianism: Text and Commentary*, and the general editor of the Prentice–Hall *Philosophy of Medicine* series.

Andrew Jameton, Ph.D., is Assistant Adjunct Professor at the Institute for Health Policy Studies, the School of Medicine, University of California, San Francisco. He is an author of a number of articles in bioethics, a coeditor of *Moral Problems in Medicine*, and the author of the forthcoming *Nursing Ethics: The Practice of Nursing and the Moral Problems of Health Care.*

John Ladd, Ph.D., is Professor of Philosophy at Brown University. He is the author of *The Structure of a Moral Code*, as well as of numerous articles in ethics and political philosophy. He is translator of Kant's *Metaphysical Elements of Justice*, the editor of *Ethical Relativism*, and the editor of *Ethical Issues Relating to Life and Death*. He is President of the American Society for Political and Legal Philosophy, and for many years was Chairman of the Committee on Philosophy and Medicine of the American Philosophical Association.

Ruth Macklin is a member of the Department of Community Health, Albert Einstein College of Medicine, Bronx. She is the author of numerous articles in ethics that have appeared in numerous journals including *Perspectives in Biology and Medicine*, is a coeditor of *Moral Problems in Medicine*, and is the author of *Man, Mind, and Morality*.

John J. Paris, S.J., Ph.D., is Associate Professor of Social Ethics, Holy Cross College, consultant in medical ethics, University of Massachusetts Medical Center, Worcester, and a member of Human Subjects Committee, St. Vincent Hospital, Worcester. He has published articles on medical ethics and on public policy in *The New England Journal of Medicine, Commonweal, Suffolk Law Review*, and elsewhere.

Seymour Perry, M.D., is on the staff of the American Association of Medical Colleges. He is the former Director, National Center for Health Care Technology, and former Assistant Surgeon General, United States Public Health Service. As an oncologist–hematologist, researcher, and administrator, Dr. Perry has published extensively in the areas of cancer research and technology assessment.

Thomas Szasz, M.D., Ph.D., is Professor of Psychiatry, Upstate Medical Center, New York. He is the author of numerous books, including *The Myth of Mental Illness, The Manufacture of Madness, Pain and Pleasure, Law, Liberty, and Psychiatry*, and *Ideology and Insanity*. An internationally known critic of many contemporary psychiatric practices, he is the cofounder of the American Association for the Abolition of Involuntary Medical Hospitalization.

ABOUT THE EDITORS

Bart Gruzalski, Ph.D., is assistant professor of philosophy and religion at Northeastern University and is codirector of the Faculty Health Care Colloquia Series at Northeastern. He writes and speaks on ethical theory and medical ethics, particularly utilitarianism, euthanasia, and the ethical issues of human and animal experimentation. His essays have appeared in a number of journals, including *Australasian Journal of Philosophy* and *Mind*, as well as in a number of anthologies. Professor Gruzalski has taught at the University of Maryland and at Bowling Green State University, and is a member of the American Philosophical Association. In 1981 he received an Excellence in Teaching Award from Northeastern University for teaching the courses "Eastern Religions" and "Philosophy of Death, Grief and Dying."

Carl Nelson, Ph.D., is associate professor and area coordinator of health care management at Northeastern University's College of Business Administration, as well as codirector of the Faculty Health Care Colloquia Series at Northeastern. He is the author of *Operations Management in the Health Services* (Elsevier–Science, forthcoming 1983) and numerous articles on the administration and delivery of services in health care organizations. Professor Nelson has taught in the management programs of the University of Manchester, Boston

University, and the Harvard School of Public Health. Professor Nelson is a member of the American Economic Association, American Association for the Advancement of Science, and the American Public Health Association. During 1982–83 he is Visiting Associate Professor of Health Systems Management at Tulane University School of Public Health and Tropical Medicine.